Transvenous Defibrillation and Radiofrequency Ablation

Edited by

A. John Camm, M.D.
Department of Cardiological Sciences
St. George's Hospital Medical School
London, United Kingdom

and

Fred W. Lindemans, Ph.D.
Medtronic
Bakken Research Center B.V.
Maastricht, The Netherlands

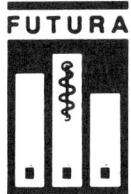

Futura Publishing
Company, Inc.
Armonk, NY

Library of Congress Cataloging-in-Publication Data
  Transvenous defibrillation and radiofrequency ablation / edited by A.
  John Camm and Fred L. Lindemans.
      p.   cm.
  Based on the symposium, New waves in arrhythmia therapies, held in
  Interlaken, Switzerland in 1993.
  Includes bibliographical references and index.
  ISBN 0-87993-605-3
  1. Implantable cardioverter–defibrillators—Congresses. 2. Catheter
  ablation—Congresses. 3. Arrhythmia—Treatment—Congresses. I. Camm,
  A. John. II. Lindemans, Frederic Willem.
  [DNLM: 1. Arrhythmia—therapy—congresses. 2. Defibrillators,
  Implantable—congresses. 3. Catheter Ablation—congresses. 4.
  Electrophysiology—congresses. WG 330 T772 1994]
  RC684.E4T73   1994
  617.4'120645—dc20
  DNLM/DLC
  for Library of Congress   94-37735
                                                                        CIP

Copyright 1995
Futura Publishing Company, Inc.

Published by
Futura Publishing Company, Inc.
135 Bedford Road
Armonk, New York 10504-0418

LC#: 94-37735
ISBN #: 0-87993-605-3

Every effort has been made to ensure that the information in this book is as up to date and as accurate as possible at the time of publication. However, due to the constant developments in medicine, neither the author, nor the editor, nor the publisher can accept any legal or any other responsibility for any errors or omissions that may occur.

All rights reserved.
No part of this book may be translated or reproduced in any form without written permission of the publisher.

Printed in the United States of America.

This book is printed on acid-free paper.

Contributors

M.A. Allessie, M.D. Department of Physiology, University of Maastricht, The Netherlands

M.H. Anderson, M.D. Department of Cardiological Sciences, St. George's Hospital Medical School, London, United Kingdom

T. Beyer, M.D. Medizinische Universitäts Klinik, Abteilung Innere Medizin III, Heidelberg, Germany

M. Block, M.D. Department of Cardiology/Angiology and Institute for Research in Arteriosclerosis, University Hospital Münster, Münster, Germany

J. Brachmann, M.D. Medizinische Universitäts Klinik, Abteilung Innere Medizin III, Heidelberg, Germany

G. Breithardt, M.D. Department of Cardiology/Angiology and Institute for Research in Arteriosclerosis, University Hospital Münster, Münster, Germany

T. Cappel, M.D. Department of Thoracic and Cardiovascular Surgery, Heinrich Heine University of Düsseldorf, Düsseldorf, Germany

Ph. Coumel, M.D. Department of Cardiology, University Hospital Lariboisière, Paris, France

A.D. Cunningham, Ph.D. Department of Pacing and Electrophysiology, Royal Brompton National Heart and Lung Hospital, London, United Kingdom

D.W. Davies, M.D. Waller Department of Cardiology, St. Mary's Hospital, London, United Kingdom

M. Di Biase, M.D. Institute of Cardiovascular Diseases, University of Bari, Bari, Italy

C.D. Dicandia, M.D. Institute of Cardiovascular Diseases, University of Bari, Bari, Italy

S. Favale, M.D.   Institute of Cardiovascular Diseases, University of Bari, Bari, Italy

B. Fischer, M.D.   Service de Cardiologie, Hôpital Saint-André, Bordeaux, France

C. Forleo, M.D.   Institute of Cardiovascular Diseases, University of Bari, Bari, Italy

M. Fromer, M.D.   Division of Cardiology, Centre Hospitalier Universitaire Vaudois, Lausanne, Switzerland

S. Hagl, M.D.   Herzchirurgische Universitäts Klinik Heidelberg, Heidelberg, Germany

M. Haissaguerre, M.D.   Service de Cardiologie, Hôpital Saint-André, Bordeaux, France

R.N.W. Hauer, M.D.   Department of Cardiology, University Hospital Utrecht, Utrecht, The Netherlands

T. Hilbel, M.D.   Medizinische Universitäts Klinik, Abteilung Innere Medizin III, Heidelberg, Germany

L. Jordaens, M.D.   Department of Cardiology, University of Gent, Gent, Belgium

W. Jung, M.D.   Department of Cardiology, University of Bonn, Bonn, Germany

L.J. Kappenberger, M.D.   Division of Cardiology, Centre Hospitalier Universitaire Vaudois, Lausanne, Switzerland

D. Keane, M.D.   Department of Interventional Cardiology, Thoraxcenter, Erasmus University, Rotterdam, The Netherlands

C.J.H.J. Kirchhof, M.D.   Department of Physiology, University of Maastricht, The Netherlands

G. Kirkorian, M.D.   Department of Cardiology, Hôpital Cardiovasculaire et Pneumologique Louis Pradel, Lyon, France

K.T.S. Konings, M.D.   Department of Physiology, University of Maastricht, The Netherlands

W. Kübler, M.D. Medizinische Universitäts Klinik, Abteilung Innere Medizin III, Heidelberg, Germany

K.-H. Kuck, M.D. Department of Cardiology, University Hospital Eppendorf, Hamburg, Germany

S. Kuhls, M.D. Department of Cardiology, Heinrich Heine University of Düsseldorf, Düsseldorf, Germany

R. Lange, M.D. Herzchirurgische Universitäts Klinik Heidelberg, Heidelberg, Germany

B. Lüderitz, M.D. Department of Cardiology, University of Bonn, Bonn, Germany

G. Luzzi, M.D. Institute of Cardiovascular Diseases, University of Bari, Bari, Italy

M. Malik, M.D. Department of Cardiological Sciences, St. George's Hospital Medical School, London, United Kingdom

G. Mannatrizio, M.D. Institute of Anaesthesiology, University of Bari, Bari, Italy

M. Manz, M.D. Department of Cardiology, University of Bonn, Bonn, Germany

H. Mehmanesh, M.D. Herzchirurgische Universitäts Klinik Heidelberg, Heidelberg, Germany

R. Mehra, Ph.D. Tachyarrhythmia Research Group, Medtronic Inc., Minneapolis, Minnesota

M. Pauschinger, M.D. Department of Cardiology, Heinrich Heine University of Düsseldorf, Düsseldorf, Germany

O.C.K.M. Penn, M.D. Department of Cardiopulmonary Surgery, University Hospital Maastricht, Maastricht, The Netherlands

C. Perings, M.D. Department of Cardiology, Heinrich Heine University of Düsseldorf, Düsseldorf, Germany

M.V. Pitzalis, M.D. Institute of Cardiovascular Diseases, University of Bari, Bari, Italy

S.G. Priori, M.D. Instituto Fisiologia Clinica e Ipertensione, University of Milan, Milan, Italy

H. Pürerfellner, M.D. Department of Cardiology, Hospital St. Elisabeth, Linz, Austria

P. Rizzon, M.D. Institute of Cardiovascular Diseases, University of Bari, Bari, Italy

E. Rowland, M.D. Department of Cardiological Sciences, St. George's Hospital Medical School, London, United Kingdom

J. Ruf-Richter Medizinische Universitäts Klinik, Abteilung Innere Medizin III, Heidelberg, Germany

R. Rüppel, M.D. Department of Cardiology, University Hospital Eppendorf, Hamburg, Germany

W. Saggau, M.D. Abteilung für Herzchirurgie, Herzzentrum Ludwigshafen, Ludwigshafen, Germany

J. Schläpfer, M.D. Division of Cardiology, Centre Hospitalier Universitaire Vaudois, Lausanne, Switzerland

M.A.E. Schneider, M.D. Department of Cardiology, University Hospital Eppendorf, Hamburg, Germany

W. Schoels, M.D. Medizinische Universitäts Klinik, Abteilung Innere Medizin III, Heidelberg, Germany

H.D. Schulte, M.D. Department of Thoracic and Cardiovascular Surgery, Heinrich Heine University of Düsseldorf, Düsseldorf, Germany

K. Seidl, M.D. Department of Cardiology, Herzzentrum Ludwigshafen, Ludwigshafen, Germany

J. Siebels, M.D. Department of Cardiology, University Hospital Eppendorf, Hamburg, Germany

J.R.L.M. Smeets, M.D. Department of Cardiology, University Hospital Maastricht, The Netherlands

L.D. Sterns, M.D. Medizinische Universitäts Klinik, Abteilung Innere Medizin III, Heidelberg, Germany

P. Tunzi, M.D. Institute of Cardiac Surgery, University of Bari, Bari, Italy

F. Veit, M.D. Department of Cardiac Surgery, Hospital of the City Vienna-Lainz, Vienna, Austria

E.G. Vester Department of Cardiology, Heinrich Heine University of Düsseldorf, Düsseldorf, Germany

J.F. Warin, M.D. Service de Cardiologie, Hôpital Saint-André, Bordeaux, France

H.J.J. Wellens, M.D. Department of Cardiology, University Hospital Maastricht, The Netherlands

J. Winter, M.D. Department of Thoracic and Cardiovascular Surgery, Heinrich Heine University of Düsseldorf, Düsseldorf, Germany

Preface

The development of the cardiac pacemaker from a historical first implant to a no longer rare medical therapy using a technically acceptable device took about a decade.

In a similar fashion, about 10 years passed between Dr. Mirowski's first human application of the automatic implantable defibrillator and the rapidly growing clinical acceptance of multi-programmable implantable cardioverter-defibrillators (ICDs) supported by indication guidelines from professional societies.

In 1991, Medtronic sponsored a symposium in Interlaken, Switzerland, in which indications, implant and follow-up techniques, clinical results of pacing and low energy cardioversion for termination of ventricular tachycardia, and other medical aspects of implantable defibrillators were presented and discussed by physicians who had participated in the clinical evaluation of new third generation ICDs. Most experience at that time had been obtained with epicardial defibrillation leads. The proceedings of this meeting were published in 1992 in Volume 5 of the Bakken Research Center Series entitled *Practical Aspects of Staged Therapy Defibrillators.**

At the second Interlaken Symposium, New Waves in Arrhythmia Therapies (1993), the program included electrophysiological aspects of atrial and ventricular fibrillation and defibrillation, results achieved with transvenous defibrillation lead systems, new indications for ICDs, and principles and practical aspects of myocardial ablation. The authors of this book have based their contributions on their presentations at this Symposium.

Although developments in the field of implantable defibrillators, with a clear trend towards pectoral implantation and extended memory functions, and in myocardial ablation, such as

---

*LJ Kappenberger, FW Lindemans: *Practical Aspects of Staged Therapy Defibrillators.* Mount Kisco, NY, Futura Publishing Co, 1992.

temperature control of the catheter tip and improved steerability, continue to be very rapid, the editors are convinced that this book will continue to be valuable for physicians interested in nonpharmacological therapies for tachyarrhythmias.

A. John Camm, M.D.
Fred W. Lindemans, Ph.D.

Acknowledgments

The task of the editors in preparing this book was easy and enjoyable because the contributors provided manuscripts that were both well prepared and, in most cases, delivered on time. We want to thank them sincerely for this and hope that they will find satisfaction in seeing their contributions in print.

We are indebted to the authors of several papers and the publishers of the various journals in which they appeared for providing permission to use some of their illustrations in this book. The sources of these figures have been indicated in the legends.

We are very grateful to Ms. Marie-Jeanne Kramer for her perseverance in preparing the materials for submission to the publisher, to Mr. Jan de Jonge for giving the finishing touch to the illustrations, and to Ms. Carla Wetzels for checking and formatting the references.

Finally, we like to thank Ms. Janet Foltin and Mr. Jacques Strauss of Futura Publishing Company for transforming a set of files and a pile of pictures into a book so quickly and Ms. Ursula Gebhardt from Medtronic for her encouragement and support.

A. John Camm, M.D.
Fred W. Lindemans, Ph.D.

Contents

Contributors iii
Preface ix
Acknowledgments xi

Chapter 1　Mapping and Pacing of Atrial Fibrillation
　　　　　　M.A. Allessie, C.J.H.J. Kirchhof, K.T.S. Konings,
　　　　　　J.R.L.M. Smeets, O.C.K.M. Penn, H.J.J. Wellens 1

Chapter 2　Mechanisms of Defibrillation
　　　　　　R. Mehra 11

Chapter 3　Electrode Configurations for Internal Atrial
　　　　　　Defibrillation
　　　　　　D. Keane 31

Chapter 4　Current Distribution around Defibrillation
　　　　　　Electrodes: Computer Modelling Approach
　　　　　　M. Malik 43

Chapter 5　Profiles of High-Risk Patients
　　　　　　G. Kirkorian 57

Chapter 6　Reflections on Guidelines for the Use of
　　　　　　Implantable Pacemaker-Cardioverter-Defibrillators
　　　　　　L.J. Kappenberger 65

Chapter 7　Which Implantable Cardioverter-Defibrillator for
　　　　　　which Patient?
　　　　　　Ph. Coumel 73

Chapter 8　Surgical Aspects of Cardioverter-Defibrillator
　　　　　　Implantation
　　　　　　F. Veit 83

Chapter 9　Influence of Electrode Position on Defibrillation
　　　　　　Threshold
　　　　　　J. Winter, C. Perings, T. Cappel, S. Kuhls,
　　　　　　M. Pauschinger, E.G. Vester, H.D. Schulte 91

Chapter 10 Implantable Transvenous Cardioverter-
Defibrillator with Pectoral Subcutaneous Patch
S. Favale, M.V. Pitzalis, G. Luzzi, C.D. Dicandia, C. Forleo,
G. Mannatrizio, P. Tunzi, M. Di Biase, P. Rizzon 99

Chapter 11 Relationship between Acute Defibrillation
Threshold and Therapy Outcome
M. Block, G. Breithardt..105

Chapter 12 Chronic Clinical Results of Nonthoracotomy
Implantable Cardioverter-Defibrillator Therapy
J. Brachmann, L.D. Sterns, T. Beyer, W. Schoels, T. Hilbel,
H. Mehmanesh, R. Lange, J. Ruf-Richter, W. Saggau,
K. Seidl, S. Hagl, W. Kübler 119

Chapter 13 Treatment of Ventricular Tachycardia with
Antitachycardia Pacing in Patients with an
Implantable Cardioverter-Defibrillator
J. Siebels, R. Rüppel, M.A.E. Schneider, K.-H. Kuck 129

Chapter 14 The Use of Antiarrhythmic Drugs in Implantable
Cardioverter-Defibrillator Patients
W. Jung, M. Manz, B. Lüderitz...137

Chapter 15 Transtelephonic Implantable Cardioverter-
Defibrillator Monitoring
M.H. Anderson..149

Chapter 16 U-CARE: Unexplained Cardiac Arrest Registry of
Europe
S.G. Priori..159

Chapter 17 Defibrillator Implantation for Patients with
Primary Electrical Disease
R.N.W. Hauer...165

Chapter 18 MIRRACLEs: A Study of Prevention of Sudden
Cardiac Death in High-Risk Patients by
Defibrillator Implantation Early after Acute
Myocardial Infarction
L. Jordaens 169

Chapter 19 The Future of Arrhythmia Surgery
O.C.K.M. Penn...177

Chapter 20 Principles and Techniques of Catheter Ablation
E. Rowland, A.D. Cunningham 187

Chapter 21	Treatment of "Mahaim" Tachycardias by Radiofrequency Catheter Ablation D.W. Davies	199
Chapter 22	Radiofrequency Ablation of the Slow Pathway in Atrioventricular Nodal Reentrant Tachycardia: Electrogram Patterns at the Successful Site B. Fischer, M. Haissaguerre, H. Pürerfellner, J.F. Warrin	209
Chapter 23	Radiation Exposure during Radiofrequency Ablation of Accessory Pathways M. Fromer, J. Schläpfer	217
Index		225

1

Mapping and Pacing of Atrial Fibrillation

M.A. Allessie, C.J.H.J. Kirchhof,
K.T.S. Konings, J.R.L.M. Smeets,
O.C.K.M. Penn, H.J.J. Wellens

This chapter addresses two different aspects of atrial fibrillation (AF). In the first part, some recent results of mapping of electrically-induced AF in man are presented.[1-5] This study has been a joint effort of the departments of physiology, cardiology, and cardiac surgery in Maastricht, The Netherlands. In the second part, some effects of local atrial pacing on the process of AF in dogs are shown.[6,7]

Atrial Fibrillation in Man

Methods and Material

The material analyzed for the first study was obtained in 25 patients undergoing surgery for the Wolff-Parkinson-White syndrome in the time that radiofrequency ablation had not yet become the therapy of choice. Seven of these patients had a history of AF, 64% were male, and the average age was 34 years, with a standard deviation of 11 years. Before starting cardiopulmonary bypass, a multi-electrode array of about 4 cm diameter was placed on the free wall of the right atrium.

From *Transvenous Defibrillation and Radiofrequency Ablation* edited by A. John Camm and Fred W. Lindemans © 1995, Futura Publishing Co., Inc., Armonk, NY.

The mapping electrode contained 248 unipolar recording electrodes with an interelectrode distance of 2.5 mm, providing the high resolution that is required for the mapping of AF.

Atrial Activation during Sinus Rhythm and Rapid Pacing

No abnormalities in atrial conduction were found during either sinus rhythm or pacing at relatively fast rates in most of these patients. Figure 1 illustrates the experimental setup and shows activation maps during sinus rhythm and during fast atrial pacing as reconstructed from the electrograms obtained from the array electrodes. Conduction is uniform and rapid, requiring about 50 ms to cover the 4 cm of the array.

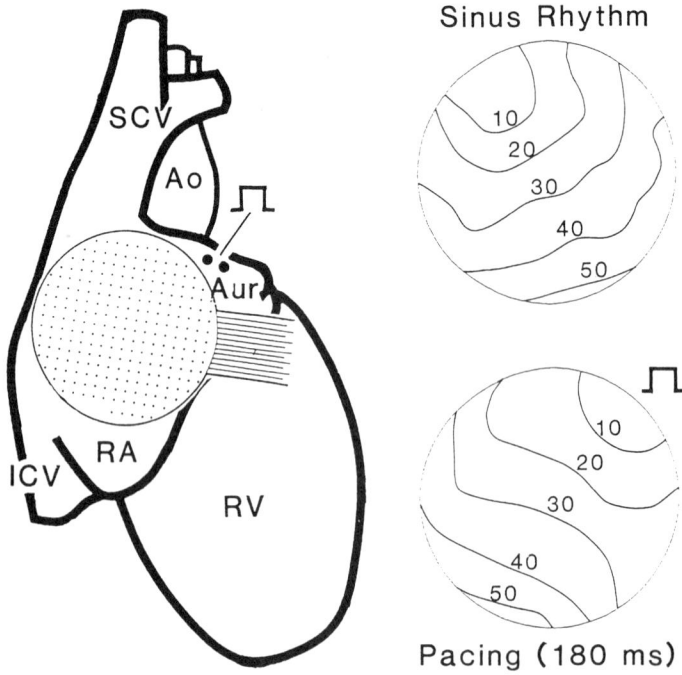

Figure 1. Left: *The multi-electrode array on the right atrial wall.* Right: *Activation isochrones obtained during sinus rhythm (top) and atrial pacing at 180 ms intervals (bottom). Reproduced with permission from Konings KTS, Kirchhof CJHJ, Smeets JRLM, et al: High density mapping of electrically induced atrial fibrillation in humans. Circulation 1994; 89:1665-1680. Copyright 1994 American Heart Association.*

Activation during Atrial Fibrillation

After these control measurements, an episode of AF was induced in each patient, either by rapid atrial pacing or by coupled extrastimuli. The episodes lasted at least a couple of minutes and only one patient required cardioversion to terminate an episode outlasting 10 minutes.

Underneath the tracing of electrocardiogram (ECG) lead III in Figure 2, confirming AF, a unipolar electrogram from one of the electrodes on the array is shown. Activation is highly irregular and rapid at this right atrial site. Pulse shape as well as cycle length vary considerably from interval to interval.

At the bottom of Figure 2, histograms of atrial and of ventricular activation are presented, illustrating the interval irregularity. The patient in this typical example had a median atrial cycle length of 140

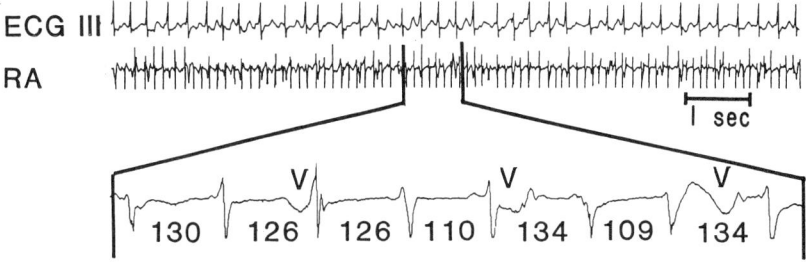

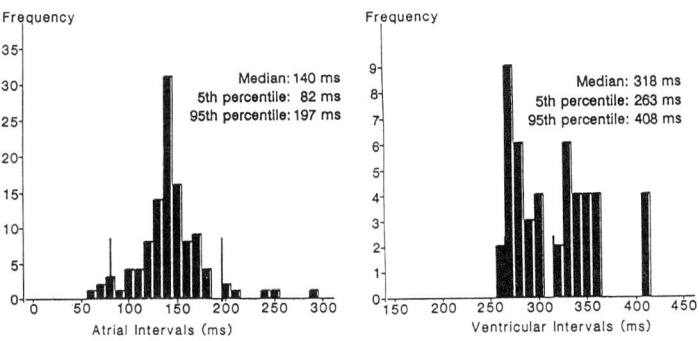

Figure 2. *Unipolar right atrial electrogram during AF (top) and atrial and ventricular interval histograms during AF (bottom). Reproduced with permission from Konings KTS, Kirchhof CJHJ, Smeets JRLM, et al: High density mapping of electrically induced atrial fibrillation in humans. Circulation 1994; 89:1665-1680. Copyright 1994 American Heart Association.*

ms, and the distance of 115 ms between the 5th and the 95th percentile illustrates the irregularity of atrial intervals.

Activation of the right atrial wall showed great differences from case to case in these patients, although surface ECGs were indistinguishable. Based on general patterns shown by the activation maps, three different types of AF were recognized: type I, type II, and type III.

During type I AF, the free wall of the right atrium is still organized in a rather regular fashion by broad excitation waves, although some areas of slow conduction or block are sometimes present. At the other end of the spectrum, during type III AF, many lines of functional conduction block are present and many different activation waves are found, all turning, reentering, and colliding. Type II AF shows intermediate patterns, varying from one big wave propagating under the array with major areas of conduction disturbances to the presence of two independent waves in that same area. These three types of AF are illustrated in Figure 3.

Figure 4 is an example of activation patterns in a patient with type I AF. Underneath ECG lead I, the figure shows a continuous right atrial electrogram recording of 12 seconds of AF. Four activation maps of the right atrial wall, with numbers referring to those underneath the electrogram, are presented. During the whole episode, activation of the right atrium is relatively uniform with one wave propagating in mainly one direction with only small beat-to-beat variations.

Three types of atrial fibrillation

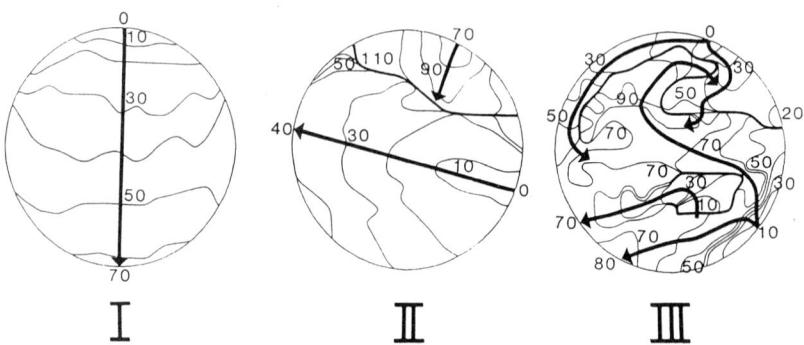

Figure 3. *The three basic patterns of atrial activation during AF are shown. Type I: Rather regular activation by one wavefront, sometimes showing small areas of slow conduction or block. Type II: One dominant excitation wave with major areas of disturbed conduction, and a second independent activation wave. Type III: Many different activation waves in chaotic pattern and many areas of conduction block.*

Mapping and Pacing of Atrial Fibrillation • 5

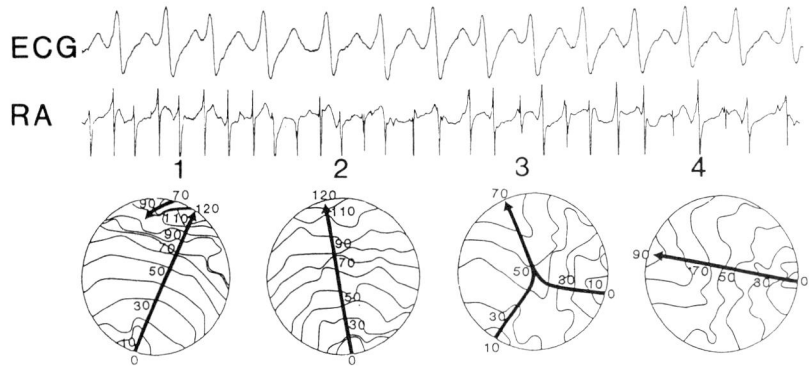

Figure 4. *ECG lead I (top) and right atrial electrogram during AF. Four activation maps, representing atrial activation at moments indicated by the numbers underneath the right atrial electrogram, show type I AF.*

Figure 5 shows how complicated activation is during type III AF. The maps show a chaotic pattern of activation with many different wavelets entering the area from various directions, turning, colliding, and extinguishing each other. By chance, one sometimes finds relatively uniform local activation with a relatively fast conduction velocity (map 4).

The results obtained in the 25 patients can be summarized below.

Type I, type II, and type III AF were present in 40%, 32%, and 28%, respectively, of the recorded maps.

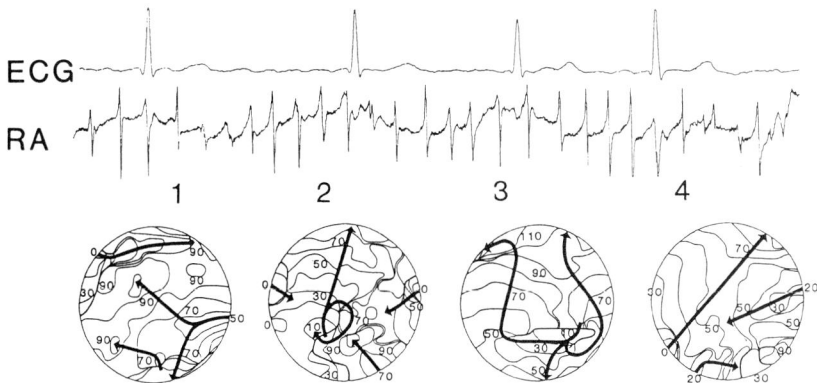

Figure 5. *ECG lead I (top) and right atrial electrogram during AF. Four activation maps, representing atrial activation at moments indicated by the numbers underneath the right atrial electrogram, show type III AF.*

Median activation intervals (±1 SD) for type I, type II, and type III AF were 174±28 ms, 147±17 ms, and 139±15 ms, respectively.

Mean interval differences between the 5th and 95th percentiles of the interval histograms were 53±25 ms, 89±23 ms, and 111±15 ms for type I, type II, and type III AF, respectively.

The percentage of time that the electrograms showed no atrial activation was 42±11, 20±4, and 7±3 for type I, type II, and type III AF, respectively.

Pace Termination of Atrial Fibrillation

The remainder of this chapter deals with the question of whether AF can be terminated by pacemaker therapy.[6,7]

Figure 6 shows a plot of atrial activation intervals during AF in a dog for 160 consecutive atrial intervals. The changes in cycle lengths

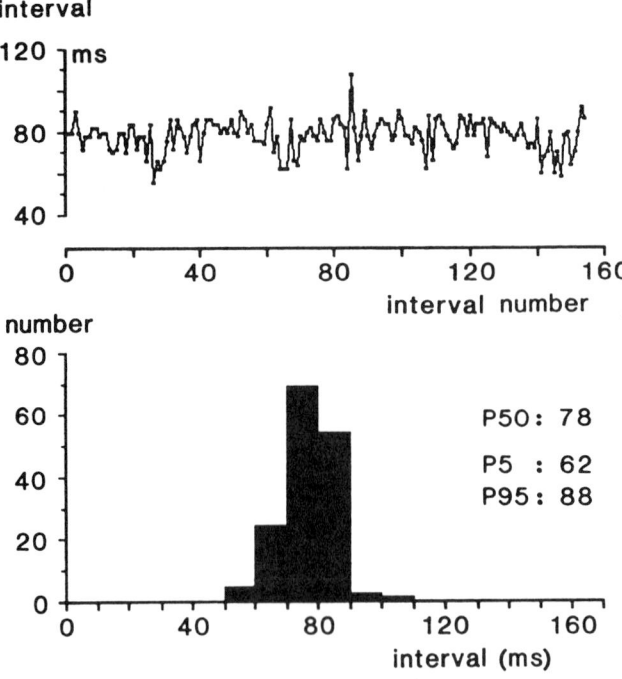

Figure 6. *160 consecutive atrial activation intervals in a dog with AF plotted by interval number (top) and shown as an interval histogram (bottom).*

are clearly visible and the intervals are presented in histogram form in the lower part of the figure.

The histogram in Figure 6 shows intervals as short as 50 to 60 ms as well as intervals as long as 70 to 110 ms. It should be possible to shorten the longer intervals by pacing. Obviously, the median cycle length during AF must be longer than the atrial refractory period.

To investigate this question further, dogs were chronically implanted with multiple electrodes on the right and left atrial wall that could be used for pacing, induction of AF, and electrogram recording. Especially in the larger dogs, induced AF can be maintained for periods up to about 30 minutes. In these chronically instrumented dogs, the possibility was tested to influence the AF process in the conscious animal by means of local stimulation.

Figure 7 shows electrograms recorded at 1, 2, and 3 cm, respectively, from the site of stimulation during AF. The amplitude of the stimuli was six times the diastolic threshold and a rather simplistic pacing pattern is used: fixed rate stimulation. At the initial part of the recordings, the stimuli clearly do not capture the atria. At the asterisk, phase lock can be observed between the stimuli and the atrial responses, which is evidence of capture. Capture is clearly evident at 1 cm and at 2 cm from the pacing site, but not at 3 cm from the pacing site.

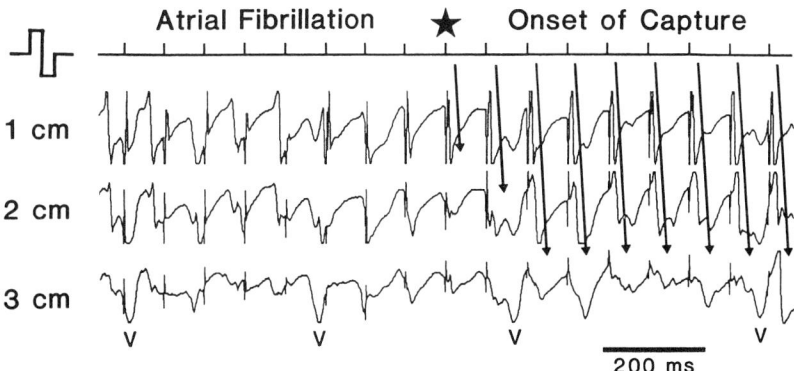

Figure 7. *Atrial electrograms recorded at 1 cm (top), 2 cm (middle), and 3 cm (bottom) from the pacing site during AF in a dog. Capture is obtained at 1 cm and 2 cm from the stimulation electrode starting at the asterisk. Reproduced with permission from Allessie MA, Kirchhof CJHJ, Scheffer GJ, et al: Regional control of atrial fibrillation by rapid pacing in conscious dogs. Circulation 1991; 84:1689-1697. Copyright 1991 American Heart Association.*

8 • TRANSVENOUS DEFIBRILLATION AND RF ABLATION

The interval window for obtaining and maintaining capture during AF is very small: for pacing intervals from 68 through 80 ms, one-to-one capture could be maintained. For pacing intervals of 67 ms or shorter and 81 ms or longer, capture could not be maintained for any significant time.

In order to further investigate how stimulation affects activation during AF, acute experiments with the previously described multi-electrode array on the left atrium of the dog were performed. Pacing was started from the center electrode of the array. The electrogram at the top of Figure 8 shows capture, starting at the arrow, during an episode of AF. Activation maps of the three beats just preceding capture

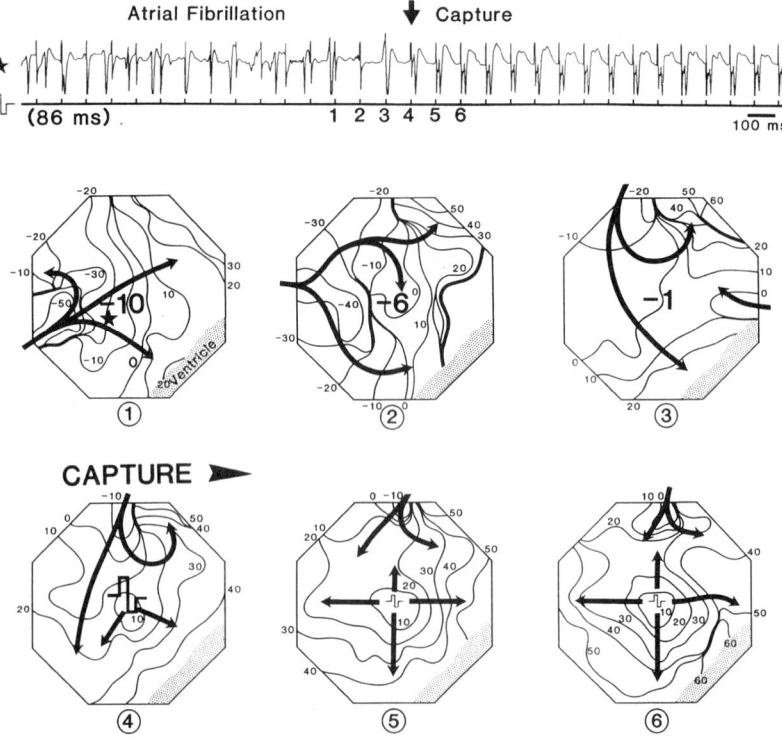

Figure 8. *Atrial electrogram in a dog with atrial pacing during AF. Capture starts at the arrow. Panels 1, 2, and 3 represent atrial activation maps before capture is obtained, panel 4 shows the activation map for the first capturing stimulus, and panels 5 and 6 show expansion of the area activated from the stimulation site. Reproduced with permission from Kirchhof CJHJ, Chorro F, Scheffer GJ, et al: Regional entrainment of atrial fibrillation studies by high-resolution mapping in open-chest dogs. Circulation 1993; 88:736-749. Copyright 1993 American Heart Association.*

and the first three beats after capture are shown underneath the electrogram tracing. When the activation wave arrives at the electrode from which pacing is performed before the stimulus is delivered, as is the case in panels 1, 2, and 3, capture cannot take place (−10, −6, and −1 at the center of the map indicate the time of arrival of the activation wave in milliseconds with respect to the timing of the stimulus). However, when the stimulus falls before arrival of a fibrillatory wave, the tissue surrounding the pacing electrodes is being activated (see panels 4, 5, and 6) and the fibrillatory wave can be pushed back by the activation started by the stimulus.

It has been possible to maintain a pattern of activation starting at the site of stimulation underneath the whole atrial area covered by the electrode array of about 4 cm diameter while AF was ongoing.

Conclusions

It has not been possible yet to terminate AF by means of overdrive pacing. It might be possible to extend the area of capture either by pacing from multiple sites or by improving the pacing mode, choosing pacing intervals more intelligently.

The appropriate timing and locations of pacing for the termination of AF should be identified, for which knowledge of the atrial refractory period might be useful. The approach of pace-termination of AF might also be combined with the use of antifibrillatory drugs or cardioversion.

References

1. Moe GK: On the multiple wavelet hypothesis of atrial fibrillation. Arch Intern Pharmacodyn 1962; 140:183-188.
2. Allessie MA, Lammers WJEP, Bonke FIM, et al: Experimental evaluation of Mow's multiple wavelet hypothesis of atrial fibrillation. In DP Zipes, J Jalife (eds.): Cardiac Arrhythmias. New York, NY, Grune & Stratton, 1985, pp. 265-276.
3. Cox JL, Canavan TE, Schuessler RB, et al: The surgical treatment of atrial fibrillation. II: Intraoperative electrophysiologic mapping and description of the electrophysiologic basis of atrial flutter and atrial fibrillation. J Thorac Cardiovasc Surg 1991; 101:406-426.
4. Wang Z, Pagé P, Nattel S: Mechanisms of flecainide's antiarrhythmic action in experimental atrial fibrillation. Circ Res 1992; 71:271-287.
5. Konings KTS, Kirchhof CJHJ, Smeets JRLM, et al: High-density mapping of electrically induced atrial fibrillation in humans. Circulation 1994; 89:1665-1680.

6. Allessie MA, Kirchhof CJHJ, Scheffer GJ, et al: Regional control of atrial fibrillation by rapid pacing in conscious dogs. Circulation 1991; 84:1689-1697.
7. Kirchhof CJHJ, Chorro F, Scheffer GJ, et al: Regional entrainment of atrial fibrillation studies by high-resolution mapping in open-chest dogs. Circulation 1993; 88:736-749.

2
Mechanisms of Defibrillation

R. Mehra

In spite of the significant advances in the technology of implantable defibrillators, the mechanism by which electrical shocks halt fibrillation is not completely understood. A better understanding of the mechanism may help reduce the defibrillation thresholds (DFTs) and the size of the implantable defibrillators. Alternatively, the longevity of the implantable cardioverter-defibrillator might be increased by the improved defibrillation technique that results from better appreciation of the defibrillation process. In this chapter, some of the experimental observations and concepts that help explain the mechanism of defibrillation are presented.

This chapter is divided into four sections. The electrophysiology of fibrillation is discussed first. Then, the basic electrophysiological effects of high voltage shocks are presented, followed by the effects of these shocks during fibrillation. Finally, these results are summarized and a hypothesis of defibrillation mechanisms is proposed.

Electrophysiology of Fibrillation

Multi-electrode mapping and computer modelling studies have given us an insight into the mechanism of fibrillation. Based on the computer simulations, Moe et al[1] proposed that fibrillation occurs as a result of multiple reentrant wavelets in the myocardium. Wavelets

From *Transvenous Defibrillation and Radiofrequency Ablation* edited by A. John Camm and Fred W. Lindemans © 1995, Futura Publishing Co., Inc., Armonk, NY.

are defined as activation wavefronts that occur due to reentry, but the path that these wavefronts traverse varies continuously and is not stable. Figure 1 illustrates the basic concept of wavelet reentry. This mechanism of fibrillation has been validated by electrical mapping studies in animals in which it was shown that multiple wavelets can exist in the heart simultaneously.[2] During atrial fibrillation, the number of wavelets changes with time and can vary between three and eight.[2] These wavelets can also occur in three dimensions.[3] Mapping during atrial fibrillation and nonsustained ventricular tachycardia (VT) has shown that spontaneous ectopic beats can also occur during these rhythms.[4] These ectopic beats are capable of retriggering tachyarrhythmias. The role that these ectopic beats play in sustaining fibrillation is unclear because computer simulations show that these wavelets can sustain fibrillation by themselves for long periods of time without the presence of ectopic beats. If these ectopic beats play a role, then the goal of defibrillation should be to stop the wavelets as well as to suppress the ectopic beats that occur spontaneously so that fibrillation is not reinitiated.

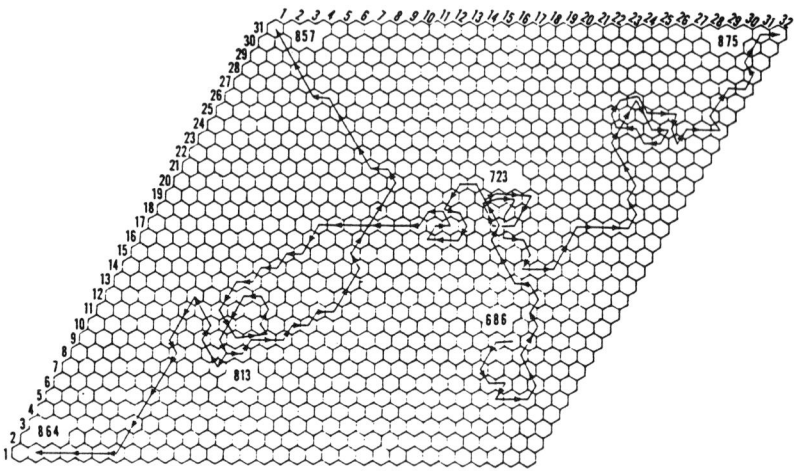

Figure 1. *The figure shows the computer generated output of conduction across a diamond shaped 31 by 32 matrix of 992 tissue-units. During fibrillation, multiple wavelets exist in the heart. Three wavelets in the upper right- and left-hand corners and one in the bottom left can be traced to a common origin at time step 686. No fixed reentrant pathways are observed and the wavelets vary in position, number, and size. Reproduced with permission from Moe GK, Rheinbolt WC, Abildskov JA: A computer model of atrial fibrillation. Am Heart J 1964; 67:200-220.*

Electrophysiological Effects of High Voltage Shocks

The effect of high voltage gradient shocks during fibrillation can be appreciated by initially understanding the effects of these shocks during rhythms that are much less complex. The electrophysiological effects of high voltage shocks delivered during paced or spontaneous sinus beats have been investigated in animal studies. The five primary effects are action potential prolongation, conduction and excitability changes, tissue damage, and postshock ectopy.

Action Potential Prolongation

Electophysiological measurements of repolarization characteristics have been made with optical methods in isolated rabbit hearts. A fiberoptic pickup is used to detect the optical signal generated by voltage-sensitive dyes that bind to cellular membrane and transduce transmembrane potential into a proportional optical signal. These recordings show that high voltage shocks prolong the action potential duration or increase the refractory period. This prolongation is dependent on the timing of the shock, its amplitude, and the waveshape. Figure 2 shows a recording made with optical methods in the rabbit ventricle.[5] The figure shows that a 10 ms duration shock coupled at 66 ms from the onset of the action potential prolongs the action potential duration by 28 ms. Prolongation has been observed with either polarity of the defibrillation shock.

In a series of canine experiments, the effect of action potential prolongation on refractory periods was also measured with electrical stimulation techniques.[6] In these studies, a band electrode was sutured around the base of the ventricle and a cup electrode was sutured around the apex of the heart. Monophasic defibrillation shocks of various amplitudes and at various coupling intervals were delivered across these two electrodes. The effective refractory period during pacing at 300 ms was measured from the center of a plaque electrode placed midway between the two defibrillation electrodes. The effective refractory period prolongation at various coupling intervals of the shock and shock amplitudes from four dogs is shown in Figure 3. The graph shows that if the shocks are delivered early in the refractory period, there is little prolongation. However, the refractory period prolongs at longer shock coupling intervals. Also, the prolongation increases with

14 • TRANSVENOUS DEFIBRILLATION AND RF ABLATION

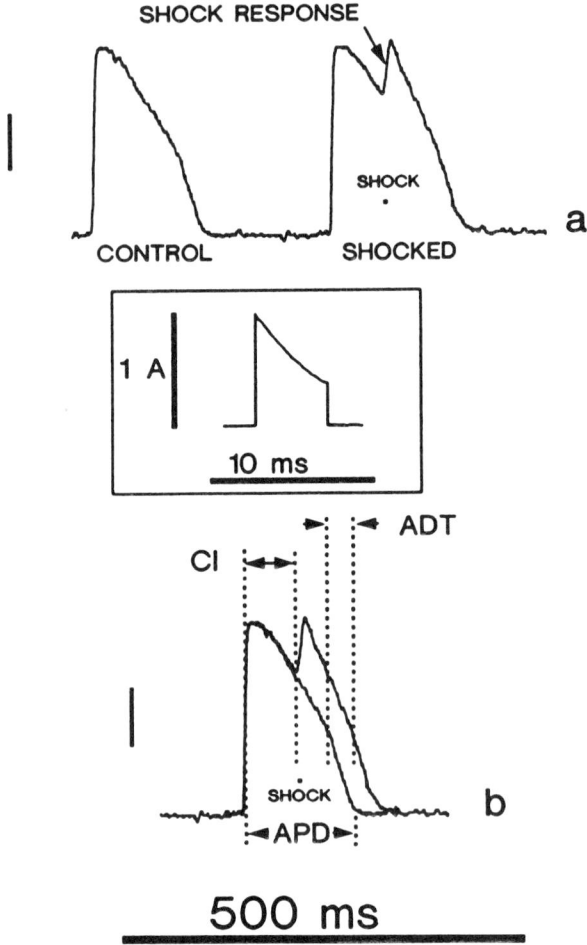

Figure 2. Tracing "a" shows a Control action potential and one receiving a 10 ms shock of 23 V/cm during repolarization. Trace "b" shows the Control and Shocked action potentials drawn over each other in order to demonstrate the disparity in the time course of their repolarization phases. The figure illustrates the shock coupling interval (CI), additional depolarization time (ADT), and the action potential duration (APD). The shock CI was 66 ms, the APD 137 ms, and the ADT 28 ms. The insert between traces "a" and "b" is the shock waveform. Reproduced from Dillon SM, Mehra R: Prolongation of ventricular refractoriness by defibrillation shocks may be due to additional depolarization of the action potential. *J Cardiovasc Electrophysiol* 1992; 3:442-456.

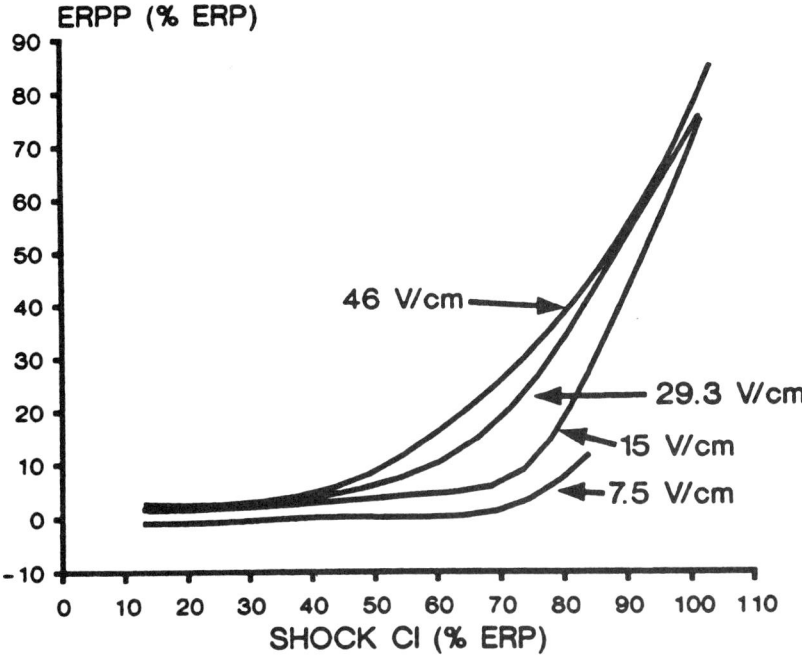

Figure 3. *Composite of the curves describing the dependence of effective refractory period prolongation (ERPP) on the shock coupling interval (CI) for four different shock gradients. Each curve is labeled by the corresponding shock voltage gradient. The ERPP and the shock CI are given as a percentage of the control effective refractory period (ERP). Reproduced from Dillon SM, Mehra R: Prolongation of ventricular refractoriness by defibrillation shocks may be due to additional depolarization of the action potential. J Cardiovasc Electrophysiol 1992; 3:442-456.*

increasing shock amplitudes. For example, when the shock is coupled at 70% of the refractory period, the prolongation is between 0% and 25% as the shock amplitude increases from 7.5 to 46 V/cm. It is important to note that a minimum gradient of 6 to 7 V/cm over most of the myocardium is required to defibrillate with a monophasic shock,[7] and the prolongation is relatively small at these gradients. At very long coupling intervals, the shock gives rise to a new propagated response, and this is reflected as a large prolongation. The same effect is also observed with biphasic shocks, although animal studies indicate that the magnitude of the prolongation is greater for monophasic than biphasic shocks and greater for longer rather than shorter durations.[8]

Conduction Changes

High voltage gradient shocks have been shown to attenuate cardiac conduction properties in animal experiments. Attenuation is observed with monophasic and biphasic shocks and the degree of attenuation is dependent on shock amplitude. Figure 4 shows the data from a study conducted by Yabe et al.[9] The heart was paced at 350 ms and a 850 V shock was delivered through a patch electrode at a coupling of 200 ms. The constant voltage gradient lines show that the voltage gradient is high close to the electrode and decreases with distance. Figure 5 shows the isochronal activation sequence due to pacing from an electrode placed in the low gradient region. Activation prior to the shock (panel A in Fig. 5) begins from the pacing electrode and traverses to the right. The first pacing beat following the shock shows conduction

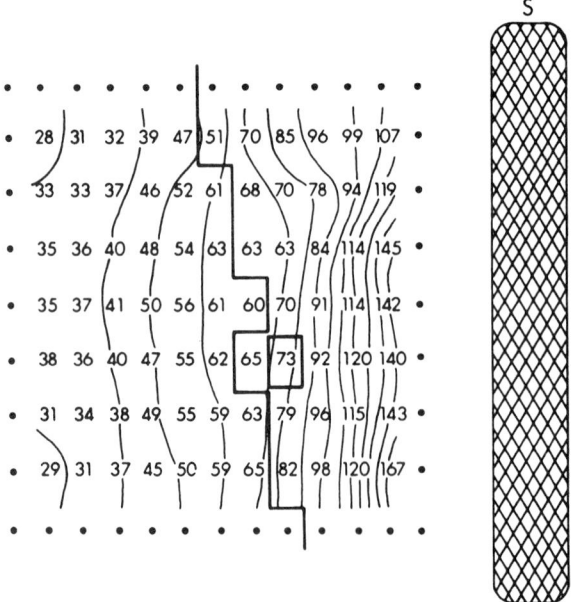

Figure 4. *Potential gradient distribution with a 850 V shock delivered between the electrode "S" on the right and an indifferent electrode. The numbers give the gradients (V/cm) and the isogradient lines are located every 10 V/cm. The wide solid line indicates the border between the region in which conduction occurred and the region in which the conduction was blocked for the first postshock cycle (see Fig. 5). Reproduced from Yabe S, Smith WM, Wolf PD, et al: Conduction disturbances caused by high current density electric fields. Circ Res 1990; 66:1190-1203. Copyright 1990 American Heart Association.*

Mechanisms of Defibrillation • 17

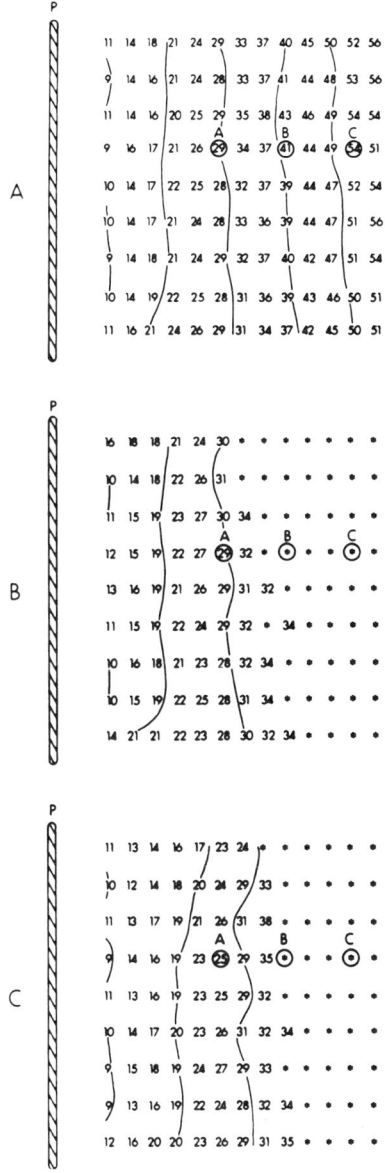

Figure 5. *Activation sequences for the preshock and first two postshock cycles. The numbers refer to local activation times in ms referenced to the beginning of the stimulus. The interval between isochronal lines is 10 ms. Panel A: The last paced cycle before the 850 V shock. Panel B: The first paced cycle after the shock. Panel C: The second paced cycle after the shock. Conduction has returned to a few of the sites that were blocked in panel A. P: pacing electrode; *: electrodes for which no activation was observed, so that conduction was considered to be blocked. Reproduced from Yabe S, Smith WM, Wolf PD, et al: Conduction disturbances caused by high current density electric fields. Circ Res 1990; 66:1190-1203. Copyright 1990 American Heart Association.*

block in the region of 60 to 70 V/cm. The conduction for the second postshock beat is improved slightly (panel C), and within 2 seconds, the conduction to that region is resumed. In the region of 100 V/cm, it takes about 5 seconds for the conduction to resume. These transient conduction changes are localized to about 1 cm from the defibrillation electrode where the gradients are high. The same effect has also been observed with biphasic shocks, but the extent of block is less. It has been hypothesized that this effect is due to the damage of the cell membranes by the high gradient shocks and changes in the intercellular coupling properties.

Excitability Changes

Increase in the pacing threshold has also been observed (following defibrillation shocks). This is probably related to a similar mechanism that causes conduction attenuation. Yee et al[10] observed that there was a 2.3-fold increase in pacing threshold when pacing was instituted immediately from the same transvenous electrode as was used for intracavitary defibrillation. This attenuation was greater at higher shock energies. The pacing threshold then decreased over the next 10 minutes, but even at the end of that period, the threshold was still higher than the control value. These changes were not observed distal to the defibrillation electrode. They postulated that the electrical injury at the interface between the catheter electrode and adjacent myocardium was the most likely explanation. Much of the electrical injury is reversible because the greatest effects are seen immediately after the shock. Pathological evidence and ST segment shifts in the ventricular electrograms support this hypothesis.

Tissue Damage

Irreversible cell damage occurs at a very high voltage gradient, probably when it is >100 V/cm. Tissue necrosis has been observed close to the electrode site in animal and clinical studies where the voltage gradients tend to be very high.[11,12] Our own animal studies indicate that the damage is significantly less with endocardial rather than epicardial patch electrodes. With epicardial electrodes, very high voltage gradients are set up in the tissue underneath the electrodes. With endocardial electrodes, the high gradient area that is localized to a few millimeters from the electrode tends to be in the intracavitary blood surrounding the catheter electrode rather than in the muscle.

Postshock Ectopic Beats

Mapping studies show that following defibrillation shocks, ectopic beats can also originate from the region of high voltage gradients close to the electrodes. In one experimental study,[9] spontaneous ectopic idioventricular beats occurred after 39% of the shocks and were more common after larger shocks. Ventricular tachycardia originating in the high gradient area near the shocking electrodes has also been observed.[13] Even in cultured myocardial cells, spontaneous postshock activation occurs following high voltage shocks.[14] This has been attributed to the "dielectric breakdown" and electromechanical deformation of the cell membranes.[14]

Effect of Shocks during Fibrillation

The electrophysiological effects of high voltage shocks during fibrillation are such that, at a critical voltage, sinus rhythm is restored. There are three critical experimental observations that have been made when high voltage shocks were delivered during fibrillation. These observations are important for elucidating the mechanism of defibrillation. They are as follows:

1. alteration of the activation pathway and early postshock reactivation in the region of the low voltage gradient following shocks that are slightly below DFT;
2. synchronization of repolarization; and
3. focal reexcitation following subthreshold defibrillation shocks.

Alteration of Activation Pathway

Several mapping studies have been conducted in animals during fibrillation. These mapping studies indicate that the process of fibrillation is due to multiple wavelets and is similar to the process observed in the computer model developed by Moe et al.[1] In the animal studies, when subthreshold defibrillation shocks were delivered, the activation maps observed following the shocks were clearly altered from those seen prior to the shock.[7,15] These results are not surprising because the tissue that is relatively refractory would become excited, whereas the tissue in the absolute refractory would undergo minimal effects. If the excitable tissue ahead of all the advancing wavefronts had been excited with sufficient prematurity by the shock, these wavefronts would be blocked and fibrillation would be terminated. Continuation of fibrillation indicates that all the original wavefronts are not extinguished or that new wavefronts are created. The probability of continuation of the original wavefronts would be highest in the region of the low voltage gradient. In experimental preparations, it was observed that the time of activation at the site of earliest reactivation after the shock was slightly later than it would have been if no shock had been given. This difference was about 10 ms, but statistically significant. Chen et al[16] have hypothesized that this occurs because the shock induces a graded response, prolongs refractoriness, and delays the activation of the next beat.

It is important to compare these results to those observed during shocks delivered in a much more organized reentrant rhythm; i.e., sustained monomorphic tachycardia.[17] Measurement of VT cycle lengths following subthreshold cardioversion shocks indicates that if progressively higher energy shocks are delivered, the VT tends to reset prior to termination; i.e., the next beat occurs earlier rather than later. This would indicate that preexcitation of excitable tissue ahead of the wavefront occurs with subthreshold cardioversion shocks. As discussed above, the data from the animal studies conducted by Chen et al[16] indicate that this is not observed following unsuccessful defibrillation shocks. One key difference between VT and ventricular fibrillation is that the basis for the former is a single reentrant circuit, while the latter is based on multiple wavelets. Why this difference would affect the relationship of the timing of the first postshock beat is unclear. Another explanation for the observations of Chen et al[16] is that in their defibrillation experiments, the resolution of the mapping electrodes may not be high enough to pick up the region of the earliest postshock excitation. Other technical factors, such as the inability of the amplifiers to record signals for a period following high energy shocks, may also account for this observation.

Reactivation in the Region of Low Gradient

Several animal studies have shown that, following a shock that is slightly below DFT, the first postshock beat is observed in the region of the low voltage gradient.[18] This indicates that all the wavefronts in the high gradient regions are extinguished and the ones in the low gradient region, although altered to some extent, continue. Figure 6 shows the results from an animal mapping study. Immediately after very low energy shocks (Fig. 6A), activations were recorded at several different sites that appeared both at the apex and base of the heart. After medium energy shocks (Fig. 6B), all activation fronts appeared to be halted in the apical half of the heart where the voltage gradient was high. Postshock activation fronts appeared in the basal half of the ventricles and fibrillation continued. Following an unsuccessful shock of 5 J (Fig. 6C), the first postshock activation beat is at the base of the heart and activations spread as large, organized fronts throughout the ventricles. This is the region of the lowest gradient because the electrodes are placed at the apex of the ventricle and on the atrial tissue. It is important to note that this is an epicardial activation map and the activations in the third dimension are not mapped. Some of the epicardial activation appears to be focal and it is possible that the intramural origin of these wavefronts are reentrant.

Synchronization of Repolarization

At any instant of time during fibrillation, the cardiac cells are in various states of repolarization.[19] This can be observed with intracellular, monophasic action potential, or optical recordings. When optical recordings are made following a high voltage shock, it is observed that the shock tends to synchronize the repolarization times of the cells as illustrated in Figure 7.[19] The figure shows the optical recordings during successive defibrillation shocks. Synchronization of repolarization occurs because the action potential is prolonged by the shock, as discussed previously. The prolongation is least for cells that are in early phase of repolarization and is maximum for those that are at later stages. The repolarization prolongation also depends on the amplitude of the voltage gradient and the shape of the shock waveform. Since most defibrillation electrodes create a nonuniform voltage gradient, this results in nonuniform prolongation, with maximum effects in the high voltage gradient areas and minimum in the low voltage region. In an ideal system, if all the cells in the heart repolarized at the same time, instant defibrillation would be observed. However, since this does not occur, the effect of action potential prolongation is to facilitate conduction block and lower the DFT. Conduction of wavefronts induced by the shock stimulus is blocked more easily because the wave-

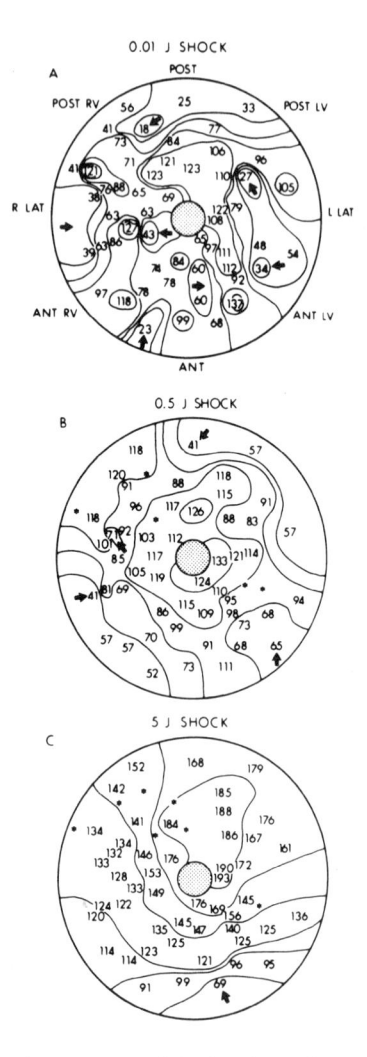

Figure 6. *Epicardial isochronal maps of the first beat after unsuccessful defibrillation shocks. A polar projection of the ventricles is shown (stippled region) with an apical electrode in the center and atrioventricular groove at periphery. Numbers represent location of electrodes with satisfactory recordings and give time of activation for those locations expressed in ms from time of onset of shock. Arrow indicates the sites of earliest postshock activation. With increasing energy, the number of early postshock sites decreased and shifted towards the base of the heart. To illustrate this effect, all tracings were aligned for the time of shock. Reproduced from Shibata N, Chen PS, Dixon EG, et al: Epicardial activation after unsuccessful defibrillation shocks in dogs. Am J Physiol 1988; 255:H902-H909.*

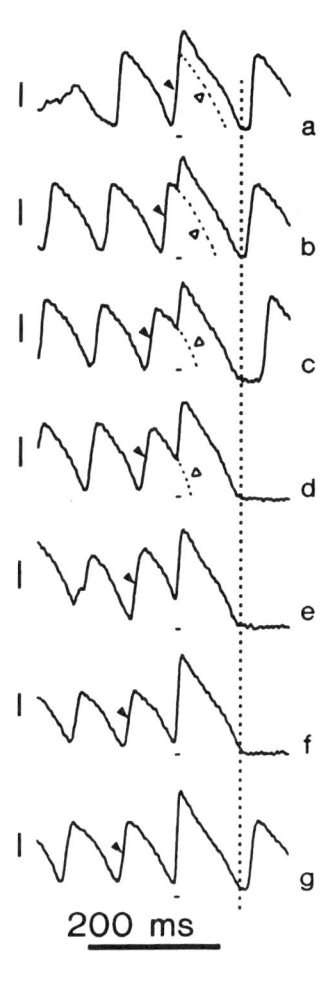

Figure 7. Optical recordings from isolated rabbit hearts obtained at a specific epicardial site during successive fibrillation episodes terminated with the same defibrillation shock energy. The shock times are indicated by thick black bars underlying traces. Filled arrowheads indicate upstroke immediately preceding shock and open arrowheads mark dashed curves showing the likely time of repolarization had the shock not been applied. Note the synchronized repolarization time following the shock as indicated by the dotted line. Reproduced from Dillon SM: Synchronized repolarization after defibrillation shocks. A possible component of the defibrillation process demonstrated by optical recordings in rabbit heart. Circulation 1992; 85:1865-1878. Copyright 1992 American Heart Association.

front confronts tissue of longer refractoriness. We tested this in a cell automata model of conduction and found that if shock-induced action potential duration prolongation was implemented in this model, its effect was primarily to reduce DFT.

Focal Reexcitation

Transient ectopic beats originating in the vicinity of the electrodes have been observed and are associated with tissue injury. In some experimental studies, however, it was observed that the first beat following an unsuccessful defibrillation shock was focal in origin and originated in the low voltage gradient area.[7,15] It is unclear whether the wavefronts appeared focal because mapping resolution was low or whether they were truly focal in origin. It is important to note that three-dimensional intramural reentry can appear focal on the epicardial surface as illustrated in Figure 8.[20] If fibrillation consists of multiple wavelets, an unsuccessful shock should either extinguish the wavefronts or alter their conduction pathway. The focal origin of postshock beats cannot be explained with this mechanism. It is possible, however,

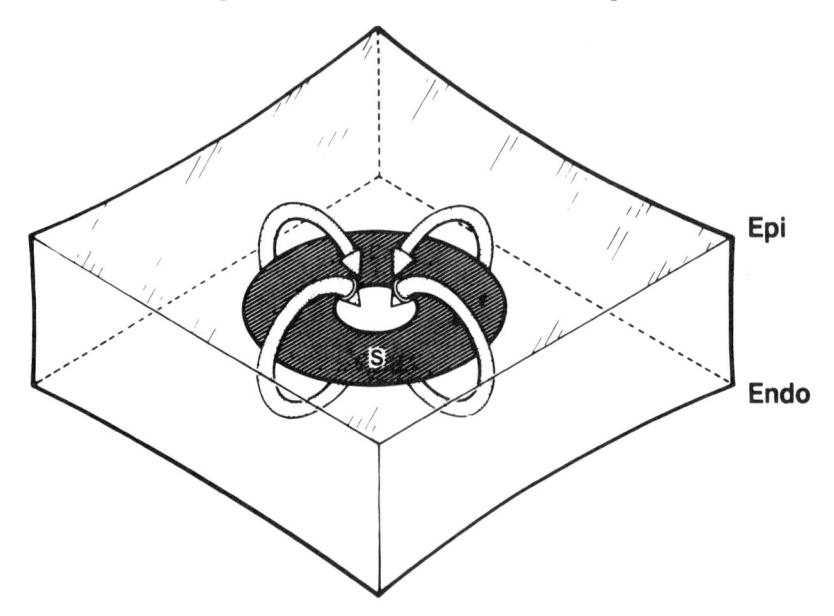

Figure 8. *Three-dimensional reentry in a block of tissue is illustrated. The reentry occurs around a toroid or doughnut (S) and the epicardial (Epi) or endocardial (Endo) maps in such a case would show focal excitation.*

that the shocks create triggered beats that are focal in origin. The other possible explanation may be that fibrillation is not totally reentrant in origin. Mapping studies in ischemic canine myocardium indicate that during unsustained VT, there are focal beats.[4] It is possible that, following a defibrillation shock, reentry is blocked, whereas the focal beats continue to reinitiate fibrillation. If this is so, then the goal of a defibrillation shock would also be to suppress ectopy.

Mechanism of Defibrillation

If the mechanism of fibrillation is the presence of multiple wavelets, then the goal of defibrillation would be to stop these wavelets and not reinitiate new wavefronts. Wavefronts are present over the whole myocardium in a fibrillating heart. At any site, the voltage gradient should be large enough to block the advancing wavefront. With an electrical stimulus of lower amplitude, excitation can occur, but it may not block the advancing wavefront. This is similar to the resetting of a VT by an electrical stimulus.[17] The fact that a reset occurs indicates that the excitable gap has been stimulated. This blocks the advancing wavefront, but the stimulus-induced wavefront continues to conduct and reentry is advanced and sustained. When the stimulus amplitude is large and sufficiently premature, the latency and prematurity of the response is short and it encounters refractory tissue ahead of it. This blocks the stimulus-induced wavefront and reentry is terminated. In fact, the basic electrophysiological mechanism of termination of fibrillation is unlikely to be very different from termination of VT by a large amplitude stimulus. The only difference between the two cases is that, in fibrillation, multiple wavefronts exist in the heart simultaneously. The key to understanding defibrillation may be an understanding of the mechanism of cardioversion.

Whether it is critically important to block *all* the wavefronts for defibrillation is not known. For example, if there were six advancing wavefronts at any time in the heart, would the heart defibrillate if all but one of these wavefronts were extinguished? The answer to this question is probably not unique and depends on the state of the remaining cardiac cells. It is reasonable to hypothesize that if all the wavefronts were blocked, defibrillation would occur. This model of defibrillation would indicate that defibrillation requires establishing an adequate voltage gradient in a critical volume of the myocardium. This critical mass may, however, be quite close to 100%, in which case its interpretation may be different than proposed originally.[21] Since

DFT is probabilistic in nature, one does not need the critical voltage gradient over the complete myocardium to defibrillate, and sometimes even lower amplitudes of shocks can be successful. This is because the spatial position of these advancing wavefronts may be such that even though the voltage gradient is inadequate in a specific region, there may not be any advancing wavefronts in that region that need to be stopped.

Mapping as well as timing studies indicate that there are changes in activation pattern with subthreshold defibrillation shocks. This could indicate that the wavefronts are "altered (reset)" or "halted and new wavefronts are reinitiated." There has been considerable debate over these two interpretations. For example, when a shock is delivered in stable reentry, reset of the tachycardia is observed. At low energies, the excitable gap may be stimulated without terminating the tachycardia. This can be interpreted as a condition in which the previously advancing wavefront was "halted and a new wavefront initiated" or as "alteration (resetting)" of the wavefronts. Either of these interpretations are compatible with the hypothesis stated previously that the goal of defibrillation is to stop the advancing wavefronts in almost all of the myocardial tissue. The only experimental observation that is incompatible with this hypothesis is the presence of postshock ectopic activation originating in the low voltage gradient region following subthreshold shocks. This represents neither the "alteration" of the wavefront nor "reinitiation of a new wavefront" that must have the properties of an advancing wavelet. Ectopic activation from the low gradient area has been observed frequently after unsuccessful defibrillation shocks.[7,15] There are three possible explanations for this occurrence. First, it is possible that the mapping resolution in these studies was inadequate and wavelet activity appeared ectopic. Second, it is possible that ectopy is normally present during fibrillation and the postshock ectopy is not shock induced but a representation of the normal fibrillation mechanism. Therefore, even if the shock stopped all advancing wavefronts, the ectopic beats would reinitiate fibrillation. This implies that, in such circumstances, the shock must also suppress ectopy to halt fibrillation. Third, the hypothesis is that the shock itself induces ectopy. The mechanism for this is not known.

The conduction and excitation changes that are observed at very high voltage gradients probably also play a role in halting all wavefronts. When a high voltage shock is delivered through an electrode, the high voltage gradient regions are close to the electrode, and fibrillation wavefronts are halted there, not only by the amplitude and prematurity of the stimulus, but also because of the increase in excitability threshold and temporary conduction block in that tissue. One observation that may be important is the initiation of focal activity at these high gradient sites that has the potential of retriggering fibrillation. As discussed previously, the role of action potential prolongation would be primarily to lower the DFT by reducing the dispersion of repolarization at adjacent sites (synchronizing repolarization), as discussed previously. If this electrophysiological mechanism was not present, defibrillation would still occur, but at a larger shock amplitude.

In the literature, two mechanisms of defibrillation have been proposed. The first one is called the "Critical Mass" and the second one is called the "Upper Limit of Vulnerability (ULV)" hypothesis. The critical mass hypothesis states that in order to defibrillate the myocardium, it is necessary to halt the fibrillation activation wavefronts in a critical mass of the muscle. The activations in the remaining mass are unable to re-engulf the ventricles into fibrillation.[22] This hypothesis is similar to that discussed above. The alternate ULV hypothesis states that unsuccessful shocks, slightly weaker than necessary to defibrillate, halt the activation fronts during fibrillation but stimulate regions of myocardium in their vulnerable period. This stimulation gives rise to new activation fronts that reinitiate fibrillation.[21] Defibrillation occurs when the shock strength is above the ULV so as not to reinduce fibrillation. This hypothesis was based on the positive correlation observed between the DFT and the upper limit of vulnerability as observed in the experimental preparations. The ULV hypothesis describes the factors that may be responsible for failure of defibrillation, but does not provide a mechanism to explain how the reinitiation of new wavefronts can be prevented to achieve defibrillation. It primarily tends to link one observational phenomenon to another.

It is still an intriguing observation that the DFT and the upper limit of vulnerability voltage are significantly correlated. This is the key observation in support of the ULV hypothesis. This indicates that, at a basic electrophysiological level, the stimulus amplitude that is required to prevent the initiation of fibrillation in sinus rhythm is correlated to that required to defibrillate. A possible explanation for this may be as follows. Fibrillation is initiated when a shock is delivered on the T wave and, due to the dispersion of repolarization, the new wavefronts conduct slowly and experience unidirectional block, and these wavelets initiate fibrillation in a manner very similar to the Moe model. However, when the shock amplitude is increased, i.e., greater than the ULV, all the excitable tissue gets activated, latency is uniformly decreased, and the probability of conduction block in all directions is increased. The same conditions exist during defibrillation. Adjacent cells in the region of the advancing wavefront are at different stages of repolarization and the electrophysiological state of the heart is not too different than during the T wave of a sinus beat. The shock stimulates the excitable tissue, blocks the advancing wavefronts and, due to the short latency of the graded response elicited by the shock, the new wavefronts are blocked. This results in defibrillation.

References

1. Moe GK, Rheinbolt WC, Abildskov JA: A computer model of atrial fibrillation. Am Heart J 1964; 67:200-220.
2. Allessie MA, Lammers WJEP, Bonke FIM, et al: Experimental evaluation of Moe's multiple wavelet hypothesis of atrial fibrillation. In DP Zipes, J Jalife (eds.): Cardiac Electrophysiology and Arrhythmias. Orlando, FL, Grune and Stratton, 1985, pp. 265-275.
3. Pogwizd SM, Corr PB: Mechanism underlying the development of ventricular fibrillation during early myocardial ischemia. Circ Res 1990; 66:404-426.
4. Pogwizd SM, Corr PB: Electrophysiologic mechanisms underlying arrhythmias due to reperfusion of ischemic myocardium. Circulation 1987; 76:404-426.
5. Dillon SM: Optical recordings in the rabbit heart show that defibrillation strength shocks prolong the duration of depolarization and the refractory period. Circ Res 1991; 69:842-856.
6. Dillon SM, Mehra R: Prolongation of ventricular refractoriness by defibrillation shocks may be due to additional depolarization of the action potential. J Cardiovasc Electrophysiol 1992; 3:442-456.
7. Zhou X, Daubert JP, Wolf PD, et al: Epicardial mapping of ventricular defibrillation with monophasic and biphasic shocks in dogs. Circ Res 1993; 72:145-160.
8. Zhou X, Wolf PD, Rollins DL, et al: Effects of monophasic and biphasic shocks on action potentials during ventricular fibrillation in dogs. Circ Res 1993; 73:325-334.
9. Yabe S, Smith WM, Wolf PD, et al: Conduction disturbances caused by high current density electric fields. Circ Res 1990; 66:1190-1203.
10. Yee R, Jones DL, Jarvis E, et al: Changes in pacing threshold and R wave amplitude after transvenous catheter countershock. J Am Coll Cardiol 1984; 4:543-549.
11. Perkins DG, Klein GJ, Silver MD, et al: Cardioversion and defibrillation using a catheter electrode: Myocardial damage assessed at autopsy. PACE 1987; 10:800-804.
12. Mower M, Mirowski M, Denniston RN, et al: The effect of intra-atrial and intraventricular countershock on the surrounding myocardium. Circulation 1971; 44:II-203.
13. Wharton JM, Wolf PD, Smith WM, et al: Cardiac potential and potential gradient fields generated by single, combined and sequential shocks during ventricular defibrillation. Circulation 1992; 85:1510-1523.

14. Jones JL, Lepeschkin E, Jones RE, et al: Response of cultured myocardial cells to countershock type electric field stimulation. Am J Physiol 1978; 235:H214-H222.
15. Chen PS, Wolf PD, Melnick SB: Comparison of activation during ventricular fibrillation and following unsuccessful defibrillation shocks in open chest dogs. Circ Res 1990; 66:1544-1553.
16. Chen PS, Wolf PD, Ideker RE: Mechanism of cardiac defibrillation. A different point of view. Circulation 1991; 84:913-919.
17. Mehra R, Prystowsky EN, Miles WM, et al: Subthreshold intracardiac cardioversion shortens ventricular tachycardia cycle length and is a predictor of cardioversion threshold. J Am Coll Cardiol 1986; 7:73A.
18. Shibata N, Chen PS, Dixon EG, et al: Epicardial activation after unsuccessful defibrillation shocks in dogs. Am J Physiol 1988; 255:H902-H909.
19. Dillon SM: Synchronized repolarization after defibrillation shocks. A possible component of the defibrillation process demonstrated by optical recordings in rabbit heart. Circulation 1992; 85:1865-1878.
20. Mehra R: Mechanism of initiation and termination of tachyarrhythmias. IEEE Eng Med Biol 1984; 34-35.
21. Chen PS, Shibata N, Dixon EG, et al: Activation during ventricular defibrillation in open chest dogs: Evidence of complete cessation and regeneration of ventricular fibrillation after unsuccessful shocks. J Clin Invest 1986; 77:810-823.
22. Zipes DP, Fisher J, King RM, et al: Termination of ventricular fibrillation in dogs by depolarizing a critical amount of myocardium. Am J Cardiol 1975; 36:35-43.
23. Walcott GP, Walcott KT, Knisley SB, et al: Mechanism of defibrillation for monophasic and biphasic waveforms. PACE 1994; 17:478-498.

3

Electrode Configurations for Internal Atrial Defibrillation

D. Keane

The development of an implantable atrial defibrillator will offer many advantages over current approaches to the management of atrial fibrillation (AF). Specifically, it should eliminate the hemodynamic embarrassment and symptoms related to rapid ventricular rates, maintain atrial systolic contribution to ventricular diastolic filling, and diminish the risk of thromboembolism. Ongoing work by Allessie's[1] group at the University of Limburg has recently demonstrated that reduction of the time spent in AF by repeated immediate cardioversion in the goat AF model may in itself prolong the duration of subsequent periods of sinus rhythm (sinus rhythm begets sinus rhythm); thus, a detraining and training effect may occur in atrial myocytes. Should such a phenomenon be shown to occur in the human atria, an implantable atrial defibrillator would be expected to offer further advantages to the patient.

In order for atrial shocks to be acceptable to the conscious patient, it is essential that an optimal electrode configuration be deployed. With the advent of the implantable ventricular defibrillator, extensive experimental and clinical research has been carried out on subcutaneous, epicardial, and endocardial electrode configurations for ventricu-

---

[1] This chapter is adapted from Kean D: Internal cardioversion of atrial arrhythmias: Review of experimental and clinical studies with implications for the design of an implantable atrial defibrillator. Eur J Cardiac Pacing Electrophysiol 1993; 4:308-314.

From *Transvenous Defibrillation and Radiofrequency Ablation* edited by A. John Camm and Fred W. Lindemans © 1995, Futura Publishing Co., Inc., Armonk, NY.

lar defibrillation. While it is unknown if the mechanism of atrial defibrillation is identical to that of ventricular defibrillation, it does seem likely that the atria and ventricles share some of the more basic principles of defibrillation. One such likely principle is that extracellular current density and potential gradient correlate closely with changes in transmembrane potentials caused by shocks and, hence, the ability to defibrillate.[2] Furthermore, it appears that a certain minimum potential gradient throughout most of the myocardium is required for defibrillation.[3] In what proportion of the atria the minimal gradient is required will depend on the atrial critical mass that remains undetermined. Tang et al[4] studied potential gradients generated by shocks delivered between a right ventricular endocardial electrode (V), a right atrial endocardial electrode (A), and a left lateral cutaneous patch (P) using a 128 electrode three-dimensional recording system in the ventricles and atria. The mean ratio of the highest to the lowest gradient was used as an index of the unevenness of the potential gradient distribution. This ratio ranged from 16.5:1 for the V + A→P electrode configuration to 26.5:1 for the V→A electrode configuration. This unevenness of the gradient field contributes to the inefficiency of ventricular defibrillation. Excessively high potential gradients (seen in the immediate proximity to intracardiac electrodes) may have deleterious effects on the myocardium and may induce conduction block and arrhythmias, while areas containing potential gradient below the "threshold gradient" may result in persistent fibrillation. Defibrillation could probably be improved by electrode configurations that produce a more even gradient field in which the minimum gradient is higher for a given shock strength. The minimum "threshold gradient" required for atrial defibrillation has yet to be determined and studies are required to study the distribution of potential gradients for exclusively atrial electrode configurations.

Electrode Configurations for Atrial Defibrillation

While much work on the optimal conditions for atrial defibrillation has yet to be conceived, a review of the results obtained from cardioversion of atrial arrhythmias in recent animal and human studies is rewarding and provides direction for future research. In view of the ease of transvenous access, most electrode configurations for internal cardioversion of atrial arrhythmias have incorporated a right atrial endocardial electrode in conjunction with either an external electrode or second right atrial electrode and, more recently, in conjunction with an intracardiac electrode in either the coronary sinus or right ventricle.

One of the early electrode configurations that combined a right atrial electrode with an external electrode for atrial defibrillation was described by Levy et al[5] who adapted the electrode configuration of conventional high energy direct current (D.C.) His bundle ablation. High energy (200 and 300 J) transcatheter cardioversion was performed by pulling back the atrioventricular junctional catheter just inferior to the site of the His bundle recording and delivering the shock between a proximal electrode (intended not to be in contact with the endocardium) and a backplate (anode). Of the 10 patients with chronic AF resistant to transthoracic shocks of up to 400 J, sinus rhythm was restored by this technique in nine patients. In a second evaluation of this high energy technique, when Kumagai et al[6] studied 10 patients with chronic lone AF, cardioversion was successful in all patients with 200 or 300 J, although one patient developed transient atrioventricular block requiring temporary pacing for 9 minutes. A subsequent randomized comparison of this technique with conventional external cardioversion in 112 patients confirmed the greater efficacy of this partly internal technique of cardioversion that achieved a 91% success rate compared to the 67% rate of conventional external cardioversion.[7]

A similar approach to internal atrial defibrillation was reported by Cotoi and colleagues[8] who combined a right atrial electrode with a precordial paddle placed on the left anterior thoracic wall (anode). This configuration was assessed in the cardioversion of four patients; two had AF and sick sinus syndrome and two had new onset AF induced by electrical stimulation of atrial flutter. Shocks of 20 J were administered without anesthesia but under sedation. Sinus rhythm was achieved in both patients with pacing-induced AF (previously atrial flutter) and transient sinus rhythm was recorded in one of the patients with chronic AF and sick sinus syndrome. Of note, in the cases in which cardioversion was successful, the right atrial electrode lay in contact with the endocardium as evidenced by the recording of monophasic action potentials. While this study involving a precordial external paddle used one tenth of the energy administered in the studies by Levy et al,[5] it is unlikely to have been a more efficacious configuration, as the success rate was poor, the study population was small, and it did not contain patients with chronic AF that had been previously resistant to conventional external cardioversion attempts. Furthermore, only the anterior wall of the right atrium lay in the high density electrical field between the two electrodes (albeit accepting that current does not flow directly within the thorax between two electrodes on account of heterogenous tissue impedances).

The right atrial catheter electrode-cutaneous patch configuration was further studied by Powell and colleagues[9] in a pace-induced AF model in sheep weighing 25 to 45 kg. Atrial defibrillation was achieved with low energies in this study by the use of an endocardial electrode of large stimulating surface area (a spring coil of 655 mm^2) and a biphasic waveform. Cardioversion occurred at a success rate of 50% (E50) at 1.5 J and 80% (E80) at 2.5 J. Eighteen (2.4%) of all 768 shocks induced ventricular fibrillation on account of T wave sensing from the surface electrocardiogram (ECG), while in a further study of 45 shocks synchronized to the right ventricular R wave, ventricular fibrillation did not occur. Of note, there was no association between the level of delivered energy and induction of ventricular fibrillation.

While configurations deploying one right atrial electrode in combination with an external electrode may achieve a higher intracardiac current density than an entirely external transthoracic system, they still involve a considerable amount of extracardiac tissue in their pathway. Thus, it is unlikely that such electrode configurations would ever be either adequately efficient or tolerable to a conscious patient. Exclusively topical (epicardial or endocardial) electrode configurations, on the other hand, might be expected to achieve higher intraatrial current densities.

Several investigators have assessed bipolar endocardial defibrillation with both electrodes positioned on a single catheter within the right atrium. In 1974, Mirowski et al[10] studied the transvenous cardioversion of atrial tachyarrhythmias in the dog. Atrial tachyarrhythmias were induced by topical acetylcholine and gentle trauma to the left atrial appendage. A bipolar defibrillating catheter was positioned in the right atrium and truncated exponential shocks were administered between a proximal electrode in the superior vena cava (SVC) and a distal electrode in the right atrium. In 125 episodes of atrial tachyarrhythmia, shocks of 0.05 to 0.5 J were usually effective, and only occasionally were 1 to 3 J required, while conversion of these tachyarrhythmias with transthoracic paddles required 40 to 100 J.

In another study of bipolar endocardial cardioversion of pace-induced atrial tachyarrhythmias in the dog, Benditt et al[11] assessed electrode catheters positioned in the right atrial appendage. Shocks of 0.16 to 1 J (rapidly decaying truncated exponential waveform) that were delivered through electrodes with a stimulating area of 20 and 26 mm^2 were universally unsuccessful, while shocks administered through electrodes with a stimulating area of 53 and 85 mm^2 did succeed intermittently, particularly when the shocks were delivered within 40 to 60 milliseconds of the preceding atrial electrogram. The overall success rate of cardioversion was 23% and, in the majority of cases, termination of the atrial tachyarrhythmia was achieved by acceleration or deceleration of atrial activity for 5 to 14 cycles, while abrupt termination with restoration of sinus rhythm occurred in the minority of successful cardioversions. In a further study by the same group, a cathodal electrode was maintained in the right atrial appendage, while three different anodal positions were compared within the right atrium: the SVC, the mid-right atrium, and the inferior vena cava.[12] Successful cardioversion was achieved at each of the three anode positions with delivered energies of ≤0.75 J, and the position of the anodal electrode within the right atrium had no consistent effect on energy requirements when the results of the dogs were combined. In this latter study, success of cardioversion was not significantly influenced by the timing of energy delivery with respect to the atrial or ventricular ECG. Timing of atrial shocks was intended to be synchronized with the atrial ECG and ventricular fibrillation was induced in 9 (2.4%) of 372 cardioversion attempts. The incidence of ventricular fibrillation induction increased with higher delivered energies; 0% at 0.01 to 0.1 J; 3.1% at 0.25 to 0.75 J; and 6.5% at energies of 1 to 5 J.

Three alternative electrode configurations in the cardioversion of atrial flutter and AF in dogs of 9 to 20 kg with talc-induced pericarditis were compared by Kumagai et al.[13] A: conventional external paddles; B: combination of a right atrial catheter electrode (cathode) and an external backplate (anode); and C: combination of a proximal and a distal electrode on a right atrial catheter. Shocks of ≤1 J resulted in successful cardioversion in 12% in configuration A, 70% in configuration B, and 74% in configuration C. Mean minimal effective energy for cardioversion was 4.0±3.52 J for configuration A, 0.62±0.67 J for configuration B, and 0.58±0.71 J for configuration C.

A bipolar, right atrial configuration was assessed in humans in a study of low energy endocardial cardioversion of a variety of arrhythmias by Nathan and colleagues.[14] Five patients studied had AF. A catheter electrode of 250 mm² surface area was placed in the right atrium in two patients and in the right ventricle in three patients. Low energy shocks (either truncated exponential or damped sinusoidal) were administered with a mean energy of 0.7 J. None of the patients with AF was converted to sinus rhythm, and one asynchronous atrial shock of 5 J resulted in ventricular fibrillation. General anesthesia was used in only one patient and sedation was given in only two. Some patients complained of severe pain with shocks of <5 J and it was felt that shocks delivered in the right atrium induced more pain than shocks delivered in the ventricle.

While the comparative study in dogs by Kumagai et al[13] demonstrated the greater efficacy of transcatheter cardioversion over conventional external cardioversion, it is unlikely that the confinement of both electrodes to the right atrium would incorporate a sufficient amount of the left atrium to be highly effective. This exclusively right atrial configuration, however, is at least as effective as the combination of a right atrial electrode with an external electrode. These studies indicate that alternative cardiac configurations (preferably with greater proximity to the left atrium) should be investigated.

Scott et al[15] evaluated two lead configurations using a right atrial J lead (RA) (7.4 cm^2), a right ventricular apical lead (RV) (5 cm^2), and two subcutaneous catheter electrodes (SQ) (6 cm^2) inserted in the 5th and 7th intercostal spaces in a study on defibrillation of the atria and ventricles in the dog. The "defibrillation threshold" using a 10 millisecond biphasic pulse was 180±63 V for the bipolar electrode configuration RV (cathode) versus RA (anode) and was 187±48 V for the tripolar configuration RV (cathode) versus RA and SQ (anode). Of interest, the defibrillation threshold of the ventricles for the latter lead configuration was 370±130 V.

In a comprehensive investigation of multiple waveforms and lead configurations in atrial defibrillation in sheep (50 to 65 kg), Cooper and colleagues[16] positioned spring coil electrodes (2.95 cm^2) in the right atrium (RA) and left pulmonary artery (LPA), a hexipolar catheter in the coronary sinus (CS), and a subcutaneous patch (133 cm^2) in the left upper chest wall (P). The optimal waveform tested was a 3/3 millisecond biphasic waveform. With this waveform, the energies associated with 50% success for the four electrode configurations were RA→P 6.9 ±1.5 J; RA→LPA 3.3±1.8 J; RA→CS+LPA 2.0±.9 J; RA→CS 1.3±.4 J. In a subsequent study by the same group, endocardial configurations in the sheep were evaluated further.[17] Electrode configurations limited to the right atrium (right→right) were compared with electrode configurations involving the right atrium and coronary sinus (right→left). All right→left configurations were more efficient than right→right configurations and the lowest 50% successful energy requirement (1.1±0.3 J) was associated with a right atrial appendage and coronary sinus combination. A recent study of endocardial cardioversion in sheep by Ayers et al[18] suggests that further reduction in energy requirements may be possible when electrodes are placed in various locations within the great cardiac vein in combination with a right atrial appendage electrode. Results of epicardial and endocardial atrial defibrillation in humans concord with the results of the Cooper et al[16,17] study, indicating that the atria can be defibrillated more effectively with a biphasic waveform than with a monophasic waveform and that endocardial cardioversion using a right atrial and coronary sinus lead configuration offers an effective system for internal atrial defibrillation.[19,20]

Electrode Polarity

In nearly all studies, the right atrial electrode was assigned to be cathodal for the delivery of shocks. The rationale for consistently administering cathodal shocks to the right atrium with the external electrode as an anode appears to have been based primarily on tradition. The only support for such an approach stems from the results of ventricular pacing studies that examined strength-interval curves for cathodal and anodal stimuli during diastole. Given, however, that during fibrillation most of the myocytes may be in a state of depolarization or incomplete repolarization,[21] and that during the relative refractory period anodal stimuli may be more effective than cathodal stimuli,[22-27] it is conceivable that lower defibrillation energy requirements may have been achieved by reversing the polarity in many of the above studies.

Effect of Electrode Location on Conduction Block

In their study of eight different electrode compositions for atrial defibrillation in the sheep, Cooper et al[17] found that sinoatrial block only occurred during shocks administered between the SVC → right atrial appendage leads, while atrioventricular block only occurred with either the low right atrium → coronary sinus or the middle right atrium → coronary sinus electrode system. Thus, not surprisingly, it appears that electrode configurations that generate high potential gradients near the sinoatrial and atrioventricular nodes are more prone to result in postshock conduction disturbances.

Effect of Electrode Location on Ventricular Arrhythmia Induction

The risk of provoking ventricular fibrillation by an asynchronous discharge is <5%.[28] The induction of ventricular fibrillation from poorly synchronized atrial shocks was reported in several of the studies on internal cardioversion described above.[9,12,14] These studies, however, used a surface ECG for R wave synchronization and no shock was reported to induce ventricular fibrillation when a direct ventricular ECG was used for synchronization.[9] A right ventricular endocardial signal, in addition to providing a reliable signal of stable amplitude, would not be prone to synchronization with high voltage repolarization waves after bandpass filtering. The intensity of electrical gradients within the ventricles resulting from low energy shocks in the atria would be expected to fall below the upper limit of vulnerability of the ventricles. Of note, in the study by Dunbar et al,[12] when both the cathodal and anodal electrodes were within the dog's right atrium, the incidence of ventricular fibrillation induction increased with the administration of shocks of higher energy. In the study by Powell and colleagues,[9] when one electrode was positioned in the sheep's right atrium and the other electrode was a lateral cutaneous patch, no association was found between delivered energy and induction of ventricular fibrillation. Cooper et al[29] reported that while no sustained ventricular arrhythmias occurred during the administration of atrial shocks that were synchronized with the R wave, episodes of nonsustained ventricular tachycardia were occasionally recorded. During testing of ventricular fibrillation induction by the administration of atrial shocks on the T wave, no difference was found between the different atrial electrode configurations and the minimum energy required to induce ventricular fibrillation (0.07±0.01 J).

The Ideal Electrode Configuration

Clearly, it is important for internal cardioversion electrode configurations to incorporate both the left as well as the right atrium within the main electrode field. Furthermore, efficiency is lost when a large amount of noncardiac tissue is included in a configuration despite the use of electrodes with large surface areas. If an electrode configuration for atrial defibrillation was designed to reduce the extracardiac dissipation of electrical energy to an absolute minimum, not only would this increase efficiency but, also, as it probably is the extracardiac energy that causes patient discomfort, such an electrode configuration would be greatly more tolerable to the conscious patient.

It is likely that the direct placement of an electrode in the left atrium in combination with a right atrial lead would lower atrial defibrillation energy requirements; however, the transseptal approach and risk of systemic thromboembolism would offset the gain in efficiency. Alternative strategies should therefore consider the placement of electrodes adjacent to the left atrium (e.g., distal coronary sinus or posterior epicardium).

Endocardial Versus Epicardial Electrode Systems

During the development of the implantable ventricular defibrillator, lead locations transgressed from initially endocardial catheters to epicardial patches and, more recently, back to endocardial catheters. For simplicity of implantation (and explantation) and pectoral placement of the device, the development of a transvenous electrode configuration for an implantable atrial defibrillator is anticipated. Should the possibility of an epicardial system for an implantable atrial defibrillator be excluded at this early stage? Unlike the implantable ventricular defibrillator, tolerance of low energy shocks from an implantable atrial defibrillator by the conscious patient will be of primary importance. It is likely that the placement of epicardial electrodes with a large electrical shadow area anteriorly over the right atrium and posteriorly over the left atrium would provide lower energy requirements for atrial defibrillation than any endocardial catheter configuration. Over the last two years, significant innovative concepts have been developed for epicardial lead design, and it will soon be possible to place epicardial electrodes with a large electrical shadow area through a small subxiphoid incision with the aid of fiberoptic pericardioscopy. The procedure will require more skill and experience than a simple transvenous implantation technique; however, the atrial shocks of lower energy and the single minimal subxiphoid incision could offer significant advantages to the patient. This may be of particular relevance if the first generation of implantable atrial defibrillators are to have backup ventricular defibrillation capabilities and the device size remains unsuitable for pectoral implantation in some patients. Thus, while an epicardial electrode system might initially appear to be unattractive to an implanting physician, the possibilities of an epicardial system should not be discarded until it has been clearly demonstrated that a transvenous endocardial system can adequately offer low atrial defibrillation energy requirements to be acceptable for all fully conscious patients.

Directions for Further Research

The planning of potential configurations might be further assisted in the future by reconstruction of intrathoracic pathways of low impedance in three-dimensional computer models[30] to provide the most homogenous distribution of charge in both atria. The impedance of electrode systems may also be reduced by the use of electrodes with large stimulating surface areas. If, however, intraatrial electrodes are excessively long, the distance between opposing electrodes becomes shorter and the possibilities for intraatrial dual pathway configurations for sequential shocks[31] may be restricted. The use of a spring coil electrode will be particularly important to maximize the electrical shadow area for a given electrode length and to avoid splinting of the coronary sinus. The French size of electrodes should be minimized to facilitate implantation through both the cephalic and subclavian veins and to avoid impedance of flow in the distal coronary sinus. Studies are required to quantify flow in the coronary sinus with electrodes of different diameter when placed in the distal coronary sinus and anterior cardiac vein. Furthermore, the value of performing coronary sinus venography (or levophase coronary sinus angiograms[32]) prior to chronic implantation of atrial defibrillation electrodes needs to be assessed.

Electrode design and location may also have to take into consideration the additional functions of sensing the ventricles as well as the atria, antibradycardia atrial pacing in the prophylaxis of vagally-mediated paroxysmal AF[33] and, possibly in the future, multipolar antitachycardia pacing in the entrainment of AF.[34] In view of the concerns for patient safety, it may be prudent to adopt a phased introduction of an implantable atrial device, initially as a dual chamber defibrillator and, subsequently, if no recordings are made of ventricular fibrillation induction, as a single chamber device.

References

1. Wijffels M, Kirchhof C, Frederiks J, et al: Atrial fibrillation begets atrial fibrillation. Circulation 1993; 88:I-18. Abstract.
2. Lepeschkin E, Jones JL, Rush S, et al: Local potential gradients as a unifying measure for thresholds of stimulation, standstill, tachyarrhythmia and fibrillation appearing after strong capacitor discharges. Adv Cardiol 1978; 21:268-278.
3. Ideker RE, Tang ASL, Frazier DW, et al: Ventricular defibrillation: Basic concepts. In N El-Sherif, P Samet (eds.): Cardiac Pacing and Electrophysiology. Philadelphia, PA, WB Saunders Co, 1991, pp. 713-726.

4. Tang AS, Wolf PW, Afework Y, et al: Three-dimensional potential gradient fields generated by intracardiac catheter and cutaneous patch electrodes. Circulation 1992; 85:1857-1864.
5. Levy S, Lacombe P, Cointe R, et al: High energy transcatheter cardioversion of chronic atrial fibrillation. J Am Coll Cardiol 1988; 12:514-518.
6. Kumagai K, Yamanouchi Y, Hiroki T, et al: Effects of transcatheter cardioversion on chronic lone atrial fibrillation. PACE 1991; 14:1571-1575.
7. Levy S, Lauribe P, Dolla E, et al: A randomised comparison of external and internal cardioversion of chronic atrial fibrillation. Circulation 1992; 86:1415-1420.
8. Cotoi S, Carasca E, Incze A, et al: Intracardiac electrical discharge in terminating atrial fibrillation. Rev Roum Physiol 1990; 27:21-24.
9. Powell A, Garan H, McGovern B, et al: Low energy conversion of atrial fibrillation in the sheep. J Am Coll Cardiol 1992; 20:707-711.
10. Mirowski M, Mower M, Langer A: Low-energy catheter cardioversion of atrial tachyarrhythmias. Clin Res 1974; 22:290A. Abstract.
11. Benditt D, Kriett J, Tobler H, et al: Cardioversion of atrial tachyarrhythmias by low energy transvenous technique. In K Steinbach (ed.): Cardiac Pacing: Proceedings of the VII World Symposium on Cardiac Pacing. Darmstadt, Germany, Steinkopff, 1982, pp. 845-851.
12. Dunbar D, Tobler G, Fetter J, et al: Intracavitary electrode catheter cardioversion of atrial tachyarrhythmias in the dog. J Am Coll Cardiol 1986; 7:1015-1027.
13. Kumagai K, Yamanouchi Y, Tashiro N, et al: Low energy synchronous transcatheter cardioversion of atrial flutter/fibrillation in the dog. J Am Coll Cardiol 1990; 16:497-501.
14. Nathan A, Bexton R, Spurrell R, et al: Internal transvenous low energy cardioversion for the treatment of cardiac arrhythmias. Br Heart J 1984; 52:377-384.
15. Scott S, Accorti P, Callaghan F, et al: Ventricular and atrial defibrillation using new transvenous tripolar and bipolar leads with 5 French electrodes and 8 French subcutaneous catheters. PACE 1991; 14(II):1893-1898.
16. Cooper R, Alferness C, Wolf P, et al: Comparison of multiple waveforms and lead configurations for internal cardioversion of atrial fibrillation in sheep. PACE 1992; 15:570. Abstract.
17. Cooper R, Alferness C, Wolf P, et al: Optimal electrode location and waveform for internal cardioversion of atrial fibrillation in sheep. Circulation 1992; 86:1791.
18. Ayers G, Ilina M, Wagner D, et al: Cardiac vein electrode locations for transvenous atrial defibrillation. J Am Coll Cardiol 1993; 21:306A. Abstract.
19. Keane D, Boyd E, Robles A, et al: Biphasic versus monophasic waveform in epicardial atrial defibrillation. PACE 1992; 15:570. Abstract.
20. Keane D, Sulke N, Cooke R, et al: Endocardial cardioversion of atrial flutter and fibrillation. PACE 1993; 4(II):928. Abstract.
21. Liem LB, Clay DA, Swerdlow CD, et al: Distinct differences in human action potential characteristics during induction of ventricular fibrillation and ventricular tachycardia. Circulation 1986; 74(suppl):II-483. Abstract.
22. Bardy GH, Ivey TD, Allen MD, et al: Evaluation of electrode polarity on defibrillation efficacy. Am J Cardiol 1989; 63:433-437.

23. O'Neill P, Boahene KA, Lawrie G, et al: The automatic implantable cardioverter-defibrillator: Effect of patch polarity on defibrillation threshold. J Am Coll Cardiol 1991; 17:707-711.
24. Mehra R, McMullen M, Furman S: Time dependence of unipolar cathodal and anodal strength-interval curves. PACE 1980; 3:526-530.
25. Mehra R, Furman S: Comparison of cathodal, anodal and bipolar strength-interval curves with temporary and permanent pacing electrodes. Br Heart J 1979; 41:468-476.
26. van Dam RT, Durrer D, Strackee J, et al: The excitability cycle of the dog's left ventricle determined by anodal, cathodal and bipolar stimulation. Circ Res 1956; IV:196-204.
27. Cranefield PF, Hoffman BF, Siebens AA: Anodal excitation of cardiac muscle. Am J Physiol 1957; 190:383-390.
28. DeSilva RA, Graboys T, Podrid PJ, et al: Cardioversion and defibrillation. Am Heart J 1980; 100:881-895.
29. Cooper R, Alferness C, Smith W, et al: Internal cardioversion of atrial fibrillation in sheep. Circulation 1993; 87:1673-1686.
30. Malik M, Smits K, Lindemans F: Effects of the anisotropic conductivity in a model of the defibrillation current density distribution. PACE 1993; 16(II):915. Abstract.
31. Keane D: Impact of pulse characteristics on atrial defibrillation energy requirements. PACE 1994; 17(2):1048-1057.
32. Haissaguerre M, Gaita F, Fischer B, et al: Radiofrequency catheter ablation of left lateral accessory pathways via the coronary sinus. Circulation 1992; 86:1464-1468.
33. Attuel P, Pellerin D, Mugica J, et al: DDD pacing: An effective treatment modality for recurrent atrial arrhythmias. PACE 1988; 11:1647-1654.
34. Kirchhof C, Chorro F, Scheffer GJ, et al: Regional entrainment of atrial fibrillation studied by high-resolution mapping in open-chest dogs. Circulation 1993; 88:736-749.

4

Current Distribution around Defibrillation Electrodes: Computer Modelling Approach

M. Malik

The accurate determinant of successful defibrillation is still the subject of electrophysiological research. However, it is generally assumed that a critical current density must be exceeded in fibrillating myocardium in order to terminate the arrhythmia.

Unfortunately, a direct measurement of the current densities within the tissues of the heart during defibrillation shocks is not possible because of serious technical and conceptual limitations. Thus, alternative approaches must be investigated in order to compare the efficacy of different defibrillation electrodes and locations prior to testing them in the clinical setting. One such possibility is computer modelling of the defibrillation shocks and computation of the myocardial current densities achieved for different positions of simulated electrodes.

A computer model of defibrillation processes may be used to guide the development of new defibrillation electrodes and, potentially, to determine optimum electrode positions in individual patients if their cardiothoracic geometry is entered into the model. For these reasons, an interest has been recently shown in mathematical and computer models of the defibrillation field and current density distribution.[1-4]

From the mathematical point of view, most of the reported models were based on the standard Laplace equation and on its solution by

From *Transvenous Defibrillation and Radiofrequency Ablation* edited by A. John Camm and Fred W. Lindemans © 1995, Futura Publishing Co., Inc., Armonk, NY.

the finite element approach.[5] However, other possibilities, such as the finite difference models,[6,7] have also been reported. As is usual with mathematical models of biomedical systems, all reported defibrillation models make several assumptions that were not entirely realistic but which are believed to be reasonable. Most frequently, these assumptions include electrically isotropic tissues and omission of insulating material implanted together with the electrodes. Many models have also been limited to only two-dimensional images of the heart or to cross-sections of the thorax.

Most of the models reported to date have been implemented on powerful mainframe or top-range mini-computers that makes their wide application not feasible. This chapter describes a model of defibrillation currents that has been implemented on a standard, i486-50 MHz powered IBM compatible personal computer. The model has been developed as an initial stage of a project aiming at forming a realistic three-dimensional model of the entire thorax that would still be implemented and operational on top-range personal computers. As the model is still under development, the version described here is only a preliminary implementation. The main goal of this chapter is to demonstrate what computer experiments are feasible and to illustrate what can be expected from more elaborate models in the future.

Description of the Model

Structure

This preliminary version of the model uses a structure of a schematized, rectangular, two-dimensional cross-section of the thorax perpendicular to the long axis of the heart (Fig. 1).

The heart is represented by an ellipsoidal region with two hollows: a circular hollow represents the left ventricular cavity while a crescent-shaped hollow represents the right ventricular cavity. These cavities are filled with blood. Outside of the heart but within the chest is the lung tissue.

In order to compare the current densities achieved during defibrillation shocks in different parts of the heart, the model distinguishes seven regions of the myocardium. Each of the left and right free ventricular walls is divided into three regions, and one region corresponds to the ventricular septum (Fig. 1).

Defibrillation Current Distribution • 45

Model structure

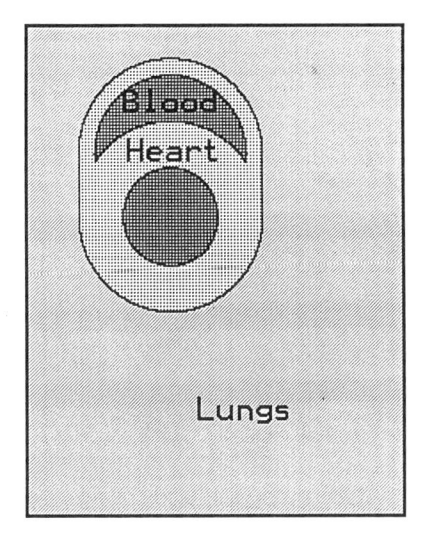

Myocardial areas

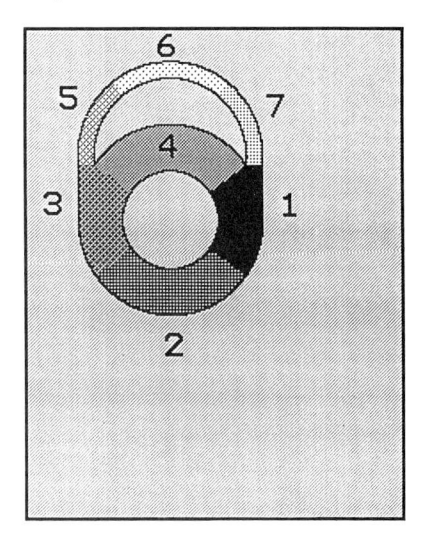

Figure 1. *The left panel shows the simplified structure of a thorax cross-section that was used in the model. The right panel shows the division of the simulated myocardial tissue into seven areas. The numbers of the areas are referred to in Figures 3 and 6 showing the samples of experimental results.*

Data of the Model

The model uses a heterogeneous structure with different electric conductivities for different tissues. In the version that was used to obtain the experiments presented in the section entitled "Samples of Computational Experiments," the ratio of (approximately) 2:6:1 was used for the conductivities of myocardium, blood (ventricular cavities), and lungs.

In principle, the model also permits the introduction of tissue anisotropy, i.e., different conductivities in different directions (e.g., along and across the bundles of myocardial fibers). This feature, however, was not used in the experiments presented here.

As the structure of the model is only a schematized image of a cross-section of the thorax, the spatial constants and the absolute values of the conductivity of individual tissues are not important. This means that the current model permits the comparison of different electrode configurations while the absolute values of current densities at individual nodes of the model (and subsequently the absolute values of cumulative current density distributions) are produced only in arbitrary technical units.

Implementation

The structure of the model was represented by a rectangular network with equidistant nodes. With the exception of those on the border of the two-dimensional structure, each node had four neighbors.

From the mathematical point of view, the potential at each node was described by a linear equation relating it to the potentials at all neighbors. The coefficients of the equations were obtained from the conductivities along the elements linking the individual nodes; the values of the coefficients were derived from the standard node form of the Kirkhoff laws. The set of equations for all nodes was solved using the standard form of Gauss-Jordan elimination.[8] The potentials at each node obtained by solving these equations and the known conductivities between neighboring nodes were used to calculate the current density at each node. This was obtained as a vector sum of currents along elements connecting the node with its neighbors.

The preliminary version of the model was implemented in three modifications with different total numbers of nodes. The experiments presented here were obtained using the largest of these modification that was composed of 66,700 nodes (rectangular network of 230 by 290 nodes).

The programs of the model were written in Turbo Pascal (Borland International). The source text of the programs, including graphics displays and evaluation routines, occupies approximately 9000 lines. The computational experiments presented here required approximately 25 MB of operating memory, and the central processing unit time demands of the model were dependent on simulated electrode positions.

Samples of Computational Experiments

Organization of Experiments

The model permits the electrodes to be placed in several regions of the simulated tissue. In more detail, the electrodes can be located at the edges of the model (subcutaneous patches), at the outer surface of the heart (epicardial patches), and in the right ventricular cavity (transvenous electrodes). The epicardial electrodes may have their outer surface electrically insulated.

The input data of individual experiments specify the location of each simulated electrode and its voltage. Positive and negative electrodes may be modelled and the voltage of each electrode can be specified within a certain range of values. Thus, intermediate electrodes with voltages between the cathode and anode can be investigated. This feature was not employed in the experiments presented here nor was the possibility of simulating a floating epicardial electrode investigated.

For each experiment, the model produces a detailed map of potentials and current densities at individual nodes. In the following sections, the maps of isocurrent-density regions are shown. In addition to these maps, the model evaluates each experiment in the terms of current density distributions in the total myocardium and in individual myocardial regions.

In order to demonstrate the capabilities of the model, two experimental series are further presented. The first series investigated the influence of the number of coils in epicardial patches. The other series inspected the influence of the position of a transvenous electrode in the right ventricular cavity in combination with a remote subcutaneous patch.

The First Experimental Set

This set of simulation experiments employed two epicardial patch electrodes with insulated outer surfaces. One of the electrodes was placed at the right ventricular free wall, the other at the left ventricular free wall. The positions of the electrodes were symmetrical in respect to the center of the schematized heart image.

While the insulated surface of each electrode was a continuous line in the two-dimensional representation, the active part of each electrode was composed of pairs of small sections that represented the coils of standard patch electrodes. The complete structure of both electrodes incorporated four coils (i.e., eight active subsections).

In each experiment of the series, the outermost coil was present in both electrodes while different combinations of the internal coils were omitted. Considering all combinations of presence and absence of the internal coils produced eight electrode configurations. All these configurations were investigated and, in each simulation experiment, the same configuration of both epicardial electrodes was used. Hence, the experimental set consisted of eight runs of the model that were subsequently compared.

Figure 2 shows the isocurrent-density maps obtained from four of the experiments. These four experiments simulated the simple com-

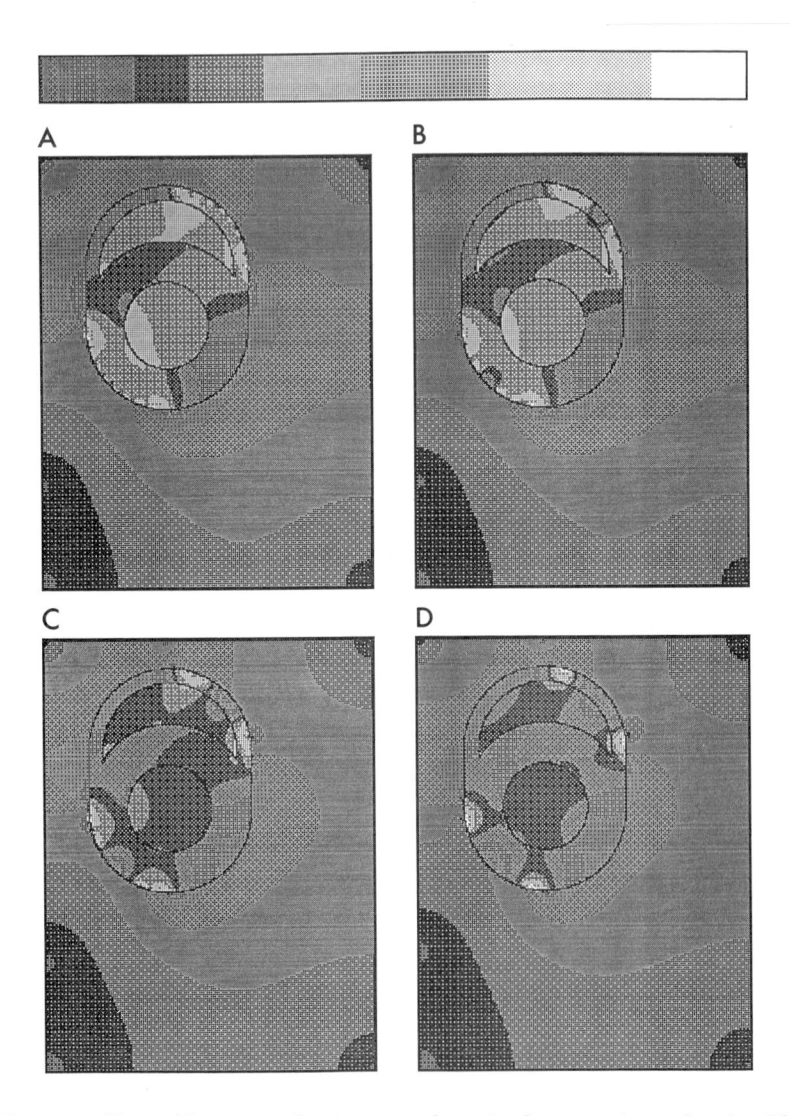

Figure 2. Plots of isocurrent-density maps from the first experimental series. The areas on the maps show the distribution of current densities on a quadratic scale that is shown on the top of the figure (the current density increases from the left to the right). Panel A shows the result of the experiment that used epicardial patches with four coils (see a more detailed description of the experimental series in the text). Panels B, C, and D show the results of experiments that used the same patches in which the central, two central, and three central coils were missing.

binations of internal coils incorporating all four, three, two, and only one outermost coil.

Figure 3 presents the cumulative current density distribution curves corresponding to all eight experiments of the series. With the exception of the experiment that simulated only the outermost coil, the cumulative current density distributions obtained for the total myocardium and for selected myocardial areas were very similar. Thus, combination of the outermost coil with any of the internal coils or any combination of the internal coils produced very similar results in terms of the current density distributions.

The Second Experimental Set

The second experimental set used a combination of a subcutaneous patch (modelled by an electrode positioned at the border of the simulated structure) with a transvenous electrode that was placed inside the right ventricular cavity. The position of the transvenous electrode was moved from one corner of the ventricular cavity to the opposite corner. Eight positions were considered between these two extremes and the total of 10 simulation experiments were performed.

Figure 4 shows the isocurrent-density maps corresponding to both extreme positions of the transvenous electrode. Figure 5 contains the cumulative current density distributions obtained from all 10 experiments for the total myocardium. It can be clearly seen that the differences between these cumulative current densities are negligible.

In spite of the close fit of the cumulative current density distributions that was obtained for the total myocardium, the cumulative current density distributions calculated for individual regions of the heart differed significantly. Figure 6 presents the cumulative current density distributions obtained from all 10 experiments for two regions of the left ventricular free wall. As these regions were symmetrical in respect to the long axis of the image of the heart, the graphs in the two panels of the figure show inverse ordering of current density plots corresponding to individual experiments. Similar observation of substantial differences between the cumulative current density distributions obtained from the 10 experiments was made also for some other myocardial regions that are not shown in Figure 6.

Discussion

The most important limitations of the current version of the model have already been mentioned. The combination of a seriously simplified structure with a restriction to a two-dimensional image does not permit the deduction of any conclusions with direct clinical applicability. Indeed, the current version of the computer model is predominantly aimed at obtaining experience with implementation of the concept on a personal computer.

Ultimately, a three-dimensional structure reflecting a substantial degree of anatomical detail should be used in conjunction with relevant data on human tissue conductivities,[9-11] including the electrical anisot-

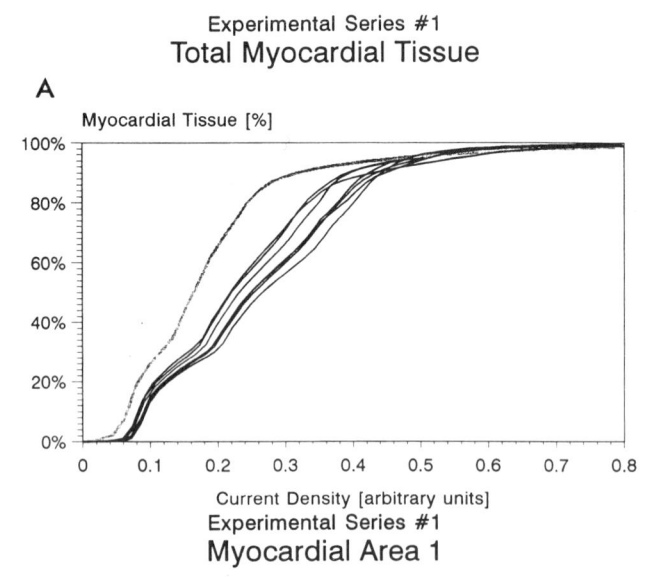

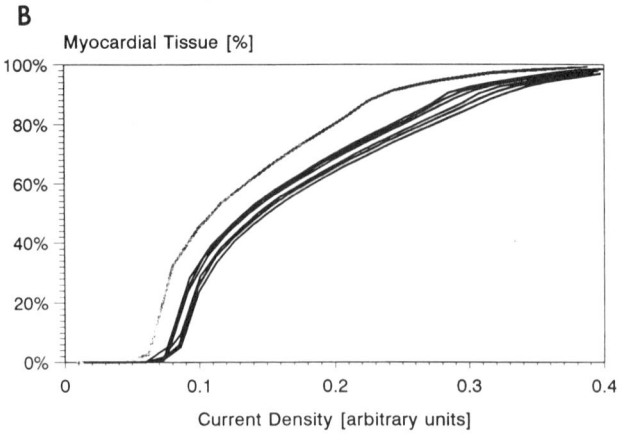

A

Experimental Series #1
Total Myocardial Tissue

B

Experimental Series #1
Myocardial Area 1

Defibrillation Current Distribution • 51

Experimental Series #1
Myocardial Area 2

C

Experimental Series #1
Myocardial Area 6

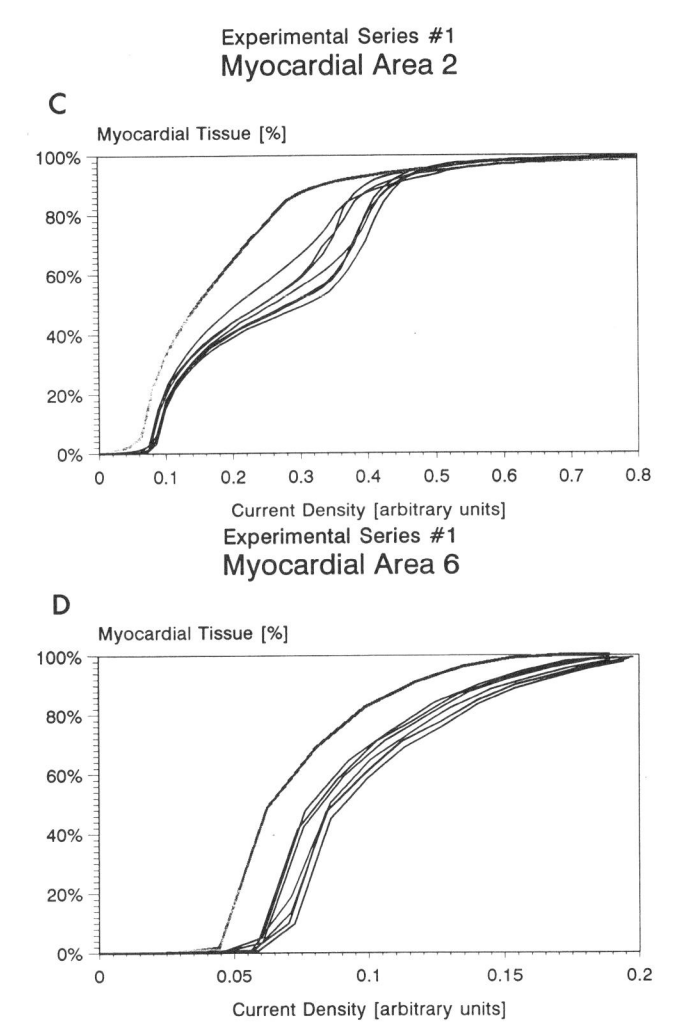

D

Figure 3. *Cumulative current density distributions derived from the first experimental series. For each experiment, the plots of the current density distributions show for each value of current density the relative amount of myocardial tissue in which the current density was lower than this value. Panel A shows the cumulative distributions for the total myocardial tissue and Panels B, C, and D show the myocardial areas 1, 2, and 6, respectively. The bold lines correspond to the experiment using only coil in the patch (see Fig. 2D); the results of all other experiments are shown in fine lines. The four panels illustrate the cumulative current density distributions for the total myocardium and for myocardial areas 1, 2, and 6, respectively (see Fig. 1).*

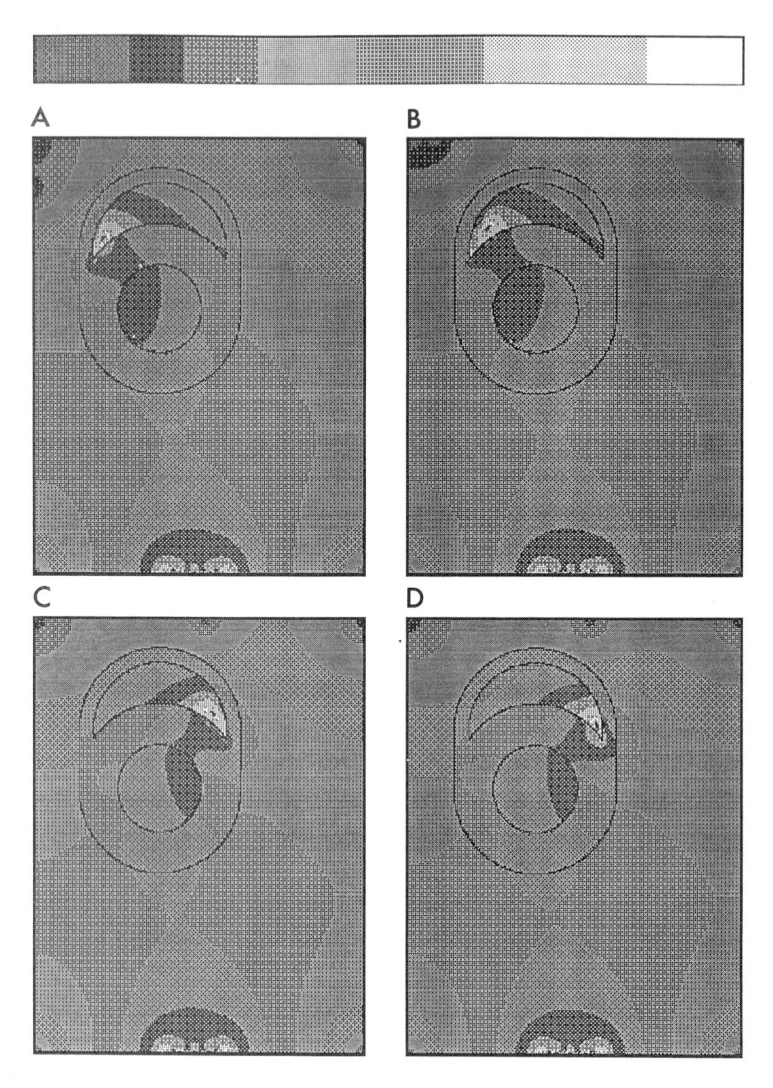

52 • TRANSVENOUS DEFIBRILLATION AND RF ABLATION

Figure 4. *Isocurrent-density maps from four experiments of the second experimental series. The areas on the maps show the distribution of current densities on a quadratic scale that is shown on the top of the figure (the current density increases from the left to the right). Panels A and B show the results of experiments placing the transvenous electrode in the left corner of the right ventricular cavity (see a more detailed description of the experimental series in the text). Panels C and D show results of experiments with the transvenous electrode in the opposite corner of the cavity.*

Experimental Series #2
Total Myocardial Tissue

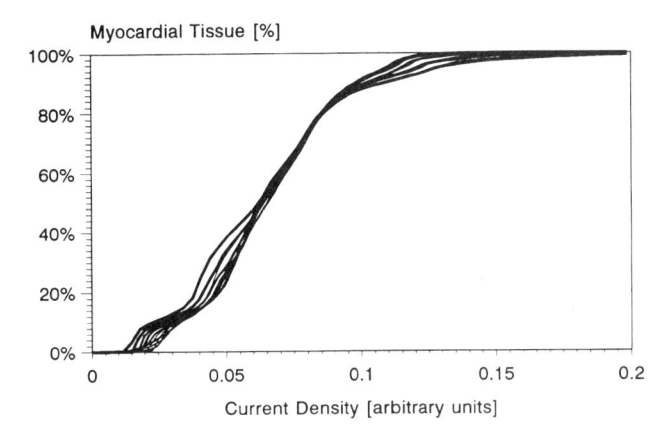

Figure 5. *Cumulative current density distributions derived from the second experimental series in total myocardium. For each experiment, plots of the current density distributions show for each value of current density the relative amount of myocardial tissue in which the current density was lower than this value. The scale of places in which the transvenous electrode was simulated is reflected by the thickness of the lines of the graphs. The very fine lines correspond to the left corner of the right ventricular cavity, and the very bold lines correspond to the right corner.*

ropy of myocardium and skeletal muscles.[12,13] Such a realistic and comprehensive model is expected to be clinically relevant; i.e., it is anticipated that computer simulation might assist the decisions on placement of defibrillation electrodes in individual patients taking into account particular cardiac pathologies.

The experience gained from experiments performed with the model described in this book will mainly be used when designing technical parameters of future models, such as the spatial constants of the grid, importance of electrical heterogeneity and anisotropy of simulated tissues, and computational efficacy of the models. Nevertheless, the experiments performed with this model might still be of practical interest. The suggestion from the first set of experiments that the number of coils in a patch electrode is not very important is worth a more detailed investigation. The other set of experiments showed that considering the cumulative current density distributions solely for the total myocardial mass does not necessarily reflect the distributions of current density achieved in specific myocardial regions.

Thus, these and similar other sets of experiments that have been carried out with the current model suggested that even intermediate

54 • TRANSVENOUS DEFIBRILLATION AND RF ABLATION

Experimental Series #2
Myocardial Area 1

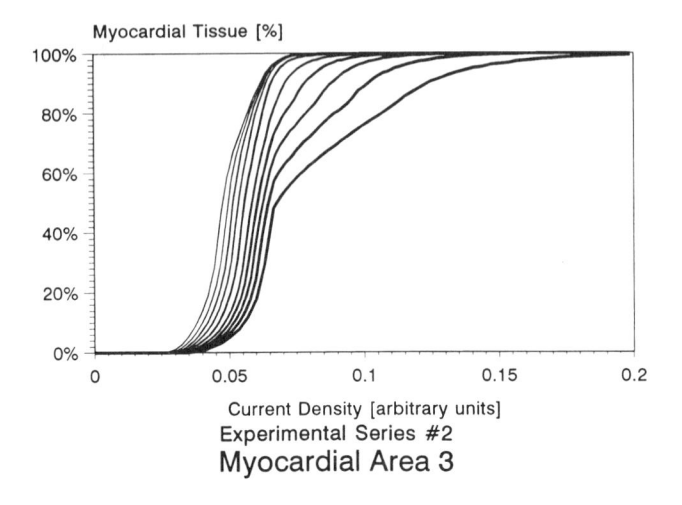

Experimental Series #2
Myocardial Area 3

Figure 6. *Cumulative current density distributions derived from the second experimental series in myocardial areas 1 and 3. For each experiment, the plots of the current density distributions show for each value of current density the relative amount of myocardial tissue in which the current density was lower than this value. The scale of places in which the transvenous electrode was simulated is reflected by the thickness of the lines of the graphs. The very fine lines correspond to the left corner of the right ventricular cavity, and the very bold lines correspond to the right corner.*

models that will not be realistic enough for modelling the characteristics of cardiac pathologies in individual patients might still provide useful technical information, e.g., suggestions for design of defibrillation electrodes.

References

1. Doian AM, Horacek BM, Rautaharju PM: Evaluation of cardiac defibrillation using a computer model of the thorax. Med Instrument 1978; 12:53-54.
2. Fahy JB, Kim Y, Ananthaswamy A: Optimal electrode configuration for external cardiac pacing and defibrillation: An inhomogeneous study. IEEE Trans Biomed Eng 1987; BME-34:743-748.
3. Barnett DW, Fahy JB, Wu H-J, et al: Finite element model applications in defibrillation and external cardiac pacing. In G Harris, C Walker (eds.): Proceedings of the Annual International Conference of the IEEE Engineering in Medicine and Biology Society. New York, NY, IEEE, 1988, pp. 200-201.
4. Sepulveda NG, Wikswo JP Jr, Echt DS: Finite element analysis of cardiac defibrillation current distributions. IEEE Trans Biomed Eng 1990; BME-37:354-365.
5. Zienkiewicz OC: The Finite Element Method. New York, NY, McGraw-Hill, 1977.
6. Hahn SJ: A flexible, interactive finite difference system for modeling defibrillation shock fields. Comput Cardiol 1992:199. Abstract.
7. Patterson R, Wang L: A finite difference model of thoracic electric fields and current flow due to surface applied defibrillation voltages. Comput Cardiol 1992:200. Abstract.
8. MacLane S, Birkhoff G: Algebra. New York, NY, Macmillan, 1968.
9. Geddes LA, Baker LE: The specific resistivity of biological material. Med Biol Eng Comput 1967; 5:271-293.
10. Van Oosterom A, de Boer RW, Van Dam RTh: Intramural resistivity of cardiac tissue. Med Biol Eng Comput 1979; 17:337-343.
11. Trautman ED, Newbower RS: A practical analysis of electrical conductivity of blood. IEEE Trans Biomed Eng 1983; BME-30:141-154.
12. Roberts DE, Tersh LT, Scher AM: Influence of cardiac fiber orientation on wavefront voltage, conduction velocity, and tissue resistivity in the dog. Circ Res 1979; 44:701-712.
13. Epstein BR, Foster KR: Anisotropy in the dielectric properties of skeletal muscle. Med Biol Eng Comput 1983; 21:51-55.

5

Profiles of High-Risk Patients

G. Kirkorian

As ventricular tachycardia (VT) and ventricular fibrillation (VF) are the most common arrhythmias documented at the time of sudden death, identification of patients at high risk for developing these arrhythmias is a prerequisite for the use of implantable cardioverter-defibrillator (ICD) therapy to prevent sudden death. It seems, therefore, appropriate to examine the current level of knowledge regarding the profile of patients at high risk of sudden cardiac death.

Patients after Myocardial Infarction

Sudden cardiac death has long been recognized as an important part of the natural history of patients recovering from an acute myocardial infarction (MI). Patients who survive have an overall mortality of about 10% during the first two years after their MI. Twenty-five percent to 50% of the deaths in this group are sudden. Table 1 summarizes the results of a number of studies dealing with mortality after MI.

The reported sudden death rates for one- to two-year follow-up periods range from 2.2% to 5% in these patients. Several factors that can be assessed prior to discharge may identify different levels of risk. Early investigators indicated that low left ventricular ejection fraction and high-grade ventricular premature beats on Holter monitoring played an important role in predicting which patients are at high risk.[1,2]

From *Transvenous Defibrillation and Radiofrequency Ablation* edited by A. John Camm and Fred W. Lindemans © 1995, Futura Publishing Co., Inc., Armonk, NY.

Table 1
Overall and Sudden Death Mortality in Post-MI Patients Reported in Some Large Series from Literature

Study	Year	Number of Patients	Follow-up (Years)	Deaths	Sudden Deaths
MPRG[1]	1983	766	2	11.0%	3.5%
MILIS[2]	1984	532	2	12.0%	5.0%
BHAT[3]	1982	1640	2	9.9%	4.6%
Kuchar[4]	1987	210	1		3.8%
Gomes[5]	1987	115	1	9.0%	4.3%
Farrell[6]	1991	416	1.7	11.3%	
Richards[7]	1991	361	2	9.4%	2.2%

Many studies have since confirmed these data. Other parameters have been added to better discriminate subgroups of patients at high risk after MI. Late potentials on the signal averaged electrogram, reduced heart rate variability, reduced baroreflex sensitivity, and arrhythmia inducibility have been claimed as the best predicting factors of arrhythmic events and/or cardiac mortality.

As an example, Richards et al[7] found in a study of 361 patients that inducibility at programmed ventricular stimulation was the best single predictor of an arrhythmic event with a relative risk (RR) of 15.2 (univariate analysis; RR = 10.4 for multivariate analysis). Good predictability with a single parameter was found also by these authors for a low ejection fraction (RR = 4.8 in univariate analysis; RR = 3.2 in multivariate analysis), large heart size (RR = 4.5), presence of late potentials (RR = 4.4), and positive Holter electrocardiogrm (ECG) (RR = 3.1).

Equally good results can be found in the literature for almost all the aforementioned parameters. How to interpret these results? It is likely that differences in patient selection, in test protocols, and in therapeutic interventions play an important role when apparently conflicting results are reported.

Two examples can help illustrate the difficulties. Table 2 shows that the proportion of patients with low ejection fraction (<40%) can vary from one study to the other: 51% of patients in the series conducted by Gomes et al[5] and around 30% for the other series. Sensitivity of low ejection fraction to predict an arrhythmic event can vary from 22% in one study to 80% in another series from the same author,[7,8] without difference in specificity. This underscores differences in patient population that seem difficult to avoid.

Table 2
Specificity and Sensitivity of Ejection Fraction below 40% as a Predictive Factor for Arrhythmic Events in Post-MI Patients

Study	Events	EF < 40%	Sensitivity	Specificity
MPRG[1]	3.5%	33%	—	—
MILIS[2]	5.0%	30%	72%	68%
Kuchar[4]	7.1%	32%	87%	74%
Gomes[5]	15.0%	52%	80%	48%
Farrell[6]	5.8%	26%	46%	75%
Farrell[8]	8.2%	—	80%	77%
Cripps[9]	9.6%	—	22%	89%
Richards[7]	4.7%	26%	71%	74%

The second example is derived from a study by Goldberg et al,[10] which showed that cardiac arrest during hospitalization for acute MI was a good predictor of survival at one year but not at five years. Clearly, the value of a predicting factor can depend on the duration of follow-up.

Many study results are presented in terms of arrhythmic events rather than cardiac arrest or sudden death. This is another limitation for interpreting these data when one tries to assess the possible reduction of mortality by ICD therapy in this setting.

In summary, low ejection fraction, late potentials, ventricular ectopy, reduced heart rate variability, reduced baroreflex sensitivity, and arrhythmia inducibility are, alone or in combination, good predictors of subsequent arrhythmic events and probably of sudden death. It is possible that a very small subgroup of patients can be identified in whom the risk of sudden death can be as high as 30% at one to two years. This percentage is an estimate that requires confirmation.

Patients with Ventricular Tachycardia

In most studies, VT and VF patients are analyzed together. It seems, however, that in a group of patients with the same etiology, incidence of sudden death is lower in the VT than in the VF group. Leclercq et al[11] reported on 295 patients with sustained monomorphic VT and without cardiac arrest, followed for an average of 61±10 months. In this series, the risk of subsequent sudden death is higher in patients with coronary heart disease or left ventricular dysfunction. The risk is negligible in patients with right heart disease or primary electrical

Table 3
Total Mortality and Sudden Death Mortality in Four Subgroups of 295 Patients with Sustained Monomorphic Ventricular Tachycardia without Arrest

Group	Overall Mortality	Sudden Death Mortality
CHD	61 (39%)	35 (22%)
LVD	15 (27%)	9 (16%)
RVD	2 (3%)	1 (2%)
no HD	0 (0%)	0 (0%)

CHD: coronary heart disease; LVD: left ventricular dysfunction; RVD: right ventricular disease; NO HD: no heart disease (primary electrical disease).
Source: Leclercq et al.[11]

disease (see Table 3). No other risk factors of sudden death have been analyzed in this paper. Thus, in a group of patients with monomorphic sustained VT, only patients with left ventricular dysfunction or coronary disease are at a relatively high risk of sudden death.

Patients with Cardiac Arrest

According to a report by Cobb et al,[12] more than 5000 victims of out-of-hospital VF have been treated in the Seattle area since 1970. Of these patients, 1162 were successfully resuscitated and discharged alive. Recurrence and survival rates have been significantly improved in these patients in recent years. Patients resuscitated during the first and second six-year period of the analysis had arrest-free survival rates of about 80%, 63%, and 52% after one, four, and eight years, respectively. Patients resuscitated during the third six-year period had 88% and 78% arrest-free survival at one and four years after the arrest, respectively. The improved rates were for recurrent cardiac arrest as well as total mortality and could not be explained. Recurrence of cardiac arrest was lower without any documented explanation, independently of ICD implantation.

The risk for recurrence of cardiac arrest could be defined by left ventricular ejection fraction at rest, history of congestive heart failure, and complex ventricular arrhythmias on ambulatory monitoring. Left ventricular function was by far the most significant predicting factor for subsequent cardiac arrest.

Even in patients at low risk of recurrent cardiac arrest, patients at a higher risk can be identified. In a retrospective survey on patients who had been discharged from the hospital alive after admission for cardiac arrest, Kudenchuk et al[13] identified 43 patients in whom left ventricular ejection fraction was higher than 50% and in whom no coronary artery stenosis was present. Seven patients (16%) had recurrent out-of-hospital cardiac arrest during a follow-up period of 86±54 months (mean±SD). The risk for recurrent cardiac arrest was 30% at five years in patients with abnormal ECGs. Recurrent cardiac arrest occurred more often among younger patients.

Electrophysiological Study Results That Can Identify Risk of Sudden Death

Independently of the nature of the ventricular arrhythmia (VT or VF), many factors can help identify patients at high risk of sudden death, among them left ventricular function and premature ventricular contractions on Holter monitoring. In addition, arrhythmia inducibility during electrophysiological study has been reported as a risk factor for subsequent cardiac arrest. Steinbeck et al[14] found that the sudden death rate after a mean follow-up of two years was 11% in patients who were noninducible at baseline and 18% in patients with an inducible arrhythmia. Furthermore, arrhythmia suppression by antiarrhythmic drugs identified patients with a more favorable outcome (sudden death rate 10%), while the sudden death rate was as high as 31% if the arrhythmia was not suppressed.

Waller et al[15] demonstrated that slowing of the induced ventricular arrhythmia and better hemodynamic tolerance in response to antiarrhythmic drugs were associated with good prognosis in terms of sudden death, despite the fact that the arrhythmia remained inducible. Patients showing this beneficial response to drug therapy had an almost identical total mortality and sudden death mortality as patients who were noninducible (see Table 4).

Actuarial analysis after three years of follow-up in these patients showed that the cumulative incidence of sudden death was about 5% for those who were either noninducible or who derived hemodynamic benefit from drug treatment and about 50% for those who had no benefit from drug treatment.

Conclusions

From this review of the literature, it can be concluded that there is no doubt that patients at highest risk of sudden death can be identified.

Table 4
Total Mortality and Sudden Death Mortality in Patients Who were Noninducible, Who Showed a Beneficial Response to Antiarrhythmic Drugs, and Who Showed No Benefit of Antiarrhythmic Drugs during Electrophysiological Testing

Group	Total Mortality	Sudden Death Mortality
Noninducible	13 (13%)	3 (3%)
Beneficial effect	6 (12%)	2 (4%)
No benefit	41 (39%)	35 (34%)

Source: Waller et al.[15]

However, to justify any intervention on the basis of risk assessment, sensitivity and specificity of the risk assessment methods must be balanced with the expected risks, benefits, and costs of the intervention.

Data from Myerburg et al[16] regarding the relative and absolute incidence of sudden death in various subgroups of the population explain why new technologies applied to the highest risk subgroups will be limited in terms of prevention of a large percentage of all sudden cardiac death cases.

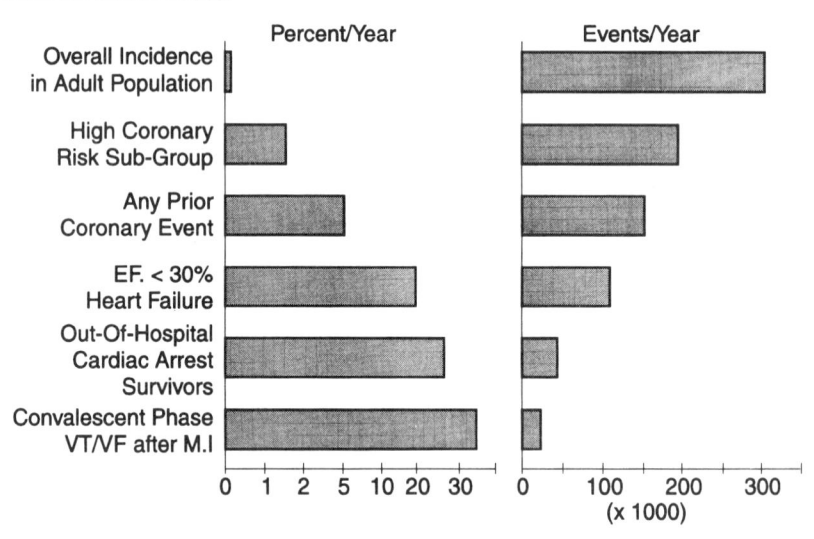

Figure 1. The risk of sudden death in percentages per year and the resulting total number of sudden death cases in various subgroups of the population. Reproduced with permission from Myerburg RJ, Kessler KM, Castellanos A: Sudden cardiac death. Structure, function, and time-dependence of risk. Circulation 1992; 85(I):2-10. Copyright 1992 American Heart Association.

As is illustrated in Figure 1, the total number of sudden death cases in population subgroups (events/year) drops substantially when subgroups with increasing relative risk are analyzed. Individuals with a high risk of sudden death constitute a relatively small proportion of the overall population at risk.

We know how to identify patients at highest risk. Whether high-risk patients are the best candidates for ICD implantation is another question.

References

1. The Multicenter Postinfarction Research Group: Risk stratification and survival after myocardial infarction. N Engl J Med 1983; 309:331-336.
2. Mukharji JM, Rude RE, Poole WK, et al: Risk factors for sudden death after acute myocardial infarction: Two-year follow-up. Am J Cardiol 1984; 54:31-36.
3. Beta-blocker Heart Attack Trial Research Group. A randomized trial of propranolol in patients with acute myocardial infarction. I. Mortality results. JAMA 1982; 247:1707-1714.
4. Kuchar DL, Thorburn CW, Sammel NL: Prediction of serious arrhythmic events after myocardial infarction: Signal-averaged electrocardiogram, Holter monitoring and radionuclide ventriculography. J Am Coll Cardiol 1987; 9:531-538.
5. Gomes JA, Winters SL, Stewart D, et al: A new non-invasive index to predict sustained ventricular tachycardia and sudden death in the first year after myocardial infarction: Based on signal-averaged electrocardiogram, radionuclide ejection fraction and Holter monitoring. J Am Coll Cardiol 1987; 10:349-357.
6. Farrell TG, Bashir Y, Cripps T, et al: Risk stratification for arrhythmic events in post infarction patients based on heart rate variability, ambulatory electrocardiographic variables and the signal-averaged electrocardiogram. J Am Coll Cardiol 1991; 18:687-697.
7. Richards DAB, Byth K, Ross DL, et al: What is the best predictor of spontaneous ventricular tachycardia and sudden death after myocardial infraction? Circulation 1991; 83:756-763.
8. Farrell TG, Odemuyiwa O, Bachir Y, et al: Prognostic value of baroreflex sensitivity testing after acute myocardial infarction. Br Heart J 1992; 67:129-137.
9. Cripps TR, Malik M, Farrell TG, et al: Prognostic value of reduced heart variability after myocardial infarction: Clinical evaluation of a new analysis method. Br Heart J 1991; 65:14-19.
10. Goldberg RJ, Gore JM, Haffajee CI, et al: Outcome after cardiac arrest during acute myocardial infarction. Am J Cardiol 1987; 59:251-255.
11. Leclercq J-F, Coumel P, Denjoy I, et al: Long-term follow-up after sustained monomorphic ventricular tachycardia: Causes, pump failure, and empiric antiarrhythmic therapy that modify survival. Am Heart J 1991; 121:1685-1692.

12. Cobb LA, Weaver D, Fahrenbruch CE, et al: Community-based intervention for sudden cardiac death. Impact, limitation and changes. Circulation 1992; 85(I):98-102.
13. Kudenchuk PJ, Cobb LA, Greene L, et al: Late outcome of survivors of out-of-hospital cardiac arrest with left ventricular ejection fractions ≥50% and without significant coronary arterial narrowing. Am J Cardiol 1991; 67:704-708.
14. Steinbeck G, Andresen D, Bach P, et al: A comparison of electrophysiologically guided antiarrhythmic drug therapy with beta-blocker therapy in patients with symptomatic, sustained ventricular tachyarrhythmias. N Engl J Med 1992; 327:987-992.
15. Waller TJ, Kay HR, Spielman SR, et al: Reduction in sudden death and mortality by antiarrhythmic therapy evaluated by electrophysiologic drug testing: Criteria of efficacy in patients with sustained ventricular tachyarrhythmia. J Am Coll Cardiol 1987; 10:83-89.
16. Myerburg RJ, Kessler KM, Castellanos A: Sudden cardiac death. Structure, function, and time-dependence of risk. Circulation 1992; 85(I):2-10.

6

Reflections on Guidelines for the Use of Implantable Pacemaker-Cardioverter-Defibrillators

L.J. Kappenberger (for the Task Force of the Working Groups on Cardiac Arrhythmias and Cardiac Pacing of the European Society of Cardiology)

Guidelines for the use of implantable defibrillators have been published by many groups.[1-4] It therefore seems absolutely unnecessary to present yet another version.

Guidelines, however, are essential for every new procedure and treatment. They resemble steps on a staircase and each reflection and improvement of the content of guidelines help to create another step up the ladder of better understanding of a therapeutic approach. Therefore, this chapter reflects on the aims, appropriateness, and the applicability of guidelines for the use of sophisticated implantable automatic antitachycardia and antifibrillatory devices. Moreover, the general applicability of such guidelines is analyzed. The main problem with guidelines that are referring to a relatively new treatment such as the implantable cardioverter-defibrillator (ICD) is that, as all the components of guidelines undergo rapid changes, the base of discussion is unstable. Within

From *Transvenous Defibrillation and Radiofrequency Ablation* edited by A. John Camm and Fred W. Lindemans © 1995, Futura Publishing Co., Inc., Armonk, NY.

a few years, technology, electrophysiological understanding, and financial resources will have changed. We further analyze how such changes might influence actual and future guidelines.

The Technology

The original implantable defibrillator was intended to terminate ventricular fibrillation (VF). Its only aim was to treat this arrhythmia and, by doing so, interrupt a cardiac arrest that might lead to sudden death. As the indication was limited to this single indication, the range of applications was rather narrow. Nevertheless, the potential of the implantable defibrillator was rapidly recognized and generally accepted. The development of a second generation of the implantable defibrillator transformed the pure defibrillator and added a cardioverter that now also could treat ventricular tachycardia (VT) with synchronized discharges. This represented tremendous progress and responded to a clinical demand after it had been shown that VF occurring in outpatient conditions was mainly the consequence of a degenerating VT.[5] But with this feature incorporated, the device could now be useful not only in a prevention of sudden death but eventually in the treatment of severe but not necessarily fatal arrhythmias.

From clinical electrophysiology, we recognized the tremendous potential of antitachycardia pacing for ventricular arrhythmias. However, the risk of acceleration prevented this technique from being used as an automatic outpatient treatment without defibrillation backup.[6] A logical combination of these ideas created the third generation of the devices referred to now as pacemaker-cardioverter-defibrillators.[7] This further step influenced again the indication. Now, treatment seems appropriate also for VTs that might not lead immediately to severe hemodynamic compromise. In fact, over 90% of arrhythmias occurring in patients with automatic implantable pacemaker-cardioverter-defibrillators are now interrupted by a sequence of pacemaker stimuli, and only in a few instances is there need for cardioversion or defibrillation shocks.[8] This makes it evident that the implantable defibrillator is not any more what it used to be.

Future developments will further influence the threshold for application of implantable defibrillator-like devices. We anticipate that tachycardia prevention might be the next step. Techniques to be applied in this situation might be: conditioning with subthreshold stimulation; arrhythmia prevention with appropriate stimulation rates; local continuous electrotonic activity to modulate conduction and automaticity; and even automatic pharmacological intervention.[9] All these future techniques will have the goal to improve the electrical stability of the heart and avoid arrhythmogenic conditions. If such features will become available, they will again be of major impact for future guidelines.

The Increase of Basic Knowledge

The development of defibrillators over the last few years has partially been in parallel with the increasing knowledge of clinical electrophysiology. Unfortunately, we have so far not been able to understand enough about the conditions leading to potentially dangerous arrhythmias in daily life. Therefore, a sort of Holter monitoring seems mandatory. So far, the Holter abilities and documentation of events with the implantable defibrillators were not extensive enough to develop substantial new insights into the origin of the serious arrhythmias and the available data have not even been analyzed fully yet. There is no information about what is happening during arrhythmia-free intervals and especially before arrhythmias appear. Our understanding of arrhythmias still results from studies performed in the electrophysiology lab and one is accustomed to extrapolating this information into patients' everyday conditions. In the clinical setting, the application of antitachycardia pacing sequences to interrupt VTs has been shown to be feasible.[10] There is still, however, a fundamental difference between an arrhythmia occurring spontaneously and an arrhythmia being provoked by programmed stimulation. It would be enormously interesting to better understand why arrhythmias occur spontaneously. In other words, devices that are as sophisticated as modern implanted defibrillators should help to increase our knowledge as to what actually happens in what I would call ambulatory electrophysiology. I anticipate fundamental differences between the results obtained in the electrophysiology laboratory compared to what is happening in daily life. In the lab, the heart is destabilized by rudely-induced unphysiological sequences of programmed ventricular stimulation, while spontaneous episodes are triggered through mechanisms not identified yet in detail and are far from being understood in principle. Much more should therefore be known about the origin of arrhythmias. New devices will have memory, but the spectrum of the information to be gained is still narrow. Guidelines must stimulate efforts for further developments and define goals for out-of-hospital arrhythmia research.

The Patient

Guidelines should define which patient at which moment benefits most from treatment. It is recommended that these guidelines are read critically. They started from the idea that the primary goal of the implantable defibrillator was to reduce sudden death from cardiac arrest induced by VF. Every documented intervention of an implantable defibrillator gives us convincing evidence that the device fulfilled this primary task. But do we really know this information on a large basis so that we can establish guidelines based on scientific facts? Unfortunately, to this day, there is no published, prospective, randomized trial to answer this question. Therefore, all of us who implant defibrillators and elaborate guidelines will do and write what they believe, based on what they see in single cases but not yet backed up by scientific and statistically acceptable data that would demonstrate in a really indisputable way its benefits and limitations. However, such information is urgently needed as there is more and more argumentation about the scientific background and the medical and human aspects of these costly interventions, especially if they are of such technical and financial impact as modern antitachycardia devices. Therefore, guidelines should help the physician to defend a therapeutic decision against financial authorities and commercial interests. Guidelines can even be considered as the legal background for a given medical procedure and, as such, can be of immense value in case of legal issues. This sword, however, has a double edge. On the one hand, the indications should be defined in a way liberal enough to leave space for individual judgment while, on the other hand, they should be strict enough to prevent abuse and to provide credible documentation for the medical profession. With this in mind, guidelines must define what is considered to be generally accepted and must, therefore, describe the conditions for which ICD implantation is warranted. To these medical reflections, financial implications have to be added that may vary from one country to another and that, unfortunately, will be sometimes the limiting factor for the choice of this treatment.

The Center

To implant a defibrillator was originally a major surgical intervention with the need for thoracotomy. This limited its use to centers with cardiothoracic surgery. Nevertheless, intraoperative mortality was quite important (up to 10%) in some centers and this mortality rate

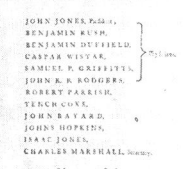

Figure 1. *A resuscitation guideline from about 1789, published by the Humane Society of Philadelphia. Courtesy of The Bakken, A Library and Museum of the Electricity in Life. Minneapolis, MN.*

had a major impact on the survival at one year.[11] Moreover, the morbidity due to an open chest intervention was high and the hospitalization period for the patients was long. As the transvenous system has now become the method of first choice, the intraoperative mortality is actually near zero and does not influence the basic patient history any longer.[12] This less difficult procedure will become even more simple with smaller units. The skill for implanting a pacemaker might one day be enough to enable a physician to implant an automatic defibrillator. Of course, we immediately fear the risk of overuse of such devices when limitation only depends on the responsibility and self-judgment of the physician. Guidelines will therefore have to define clearly who should implant an automatic defibrillator and where this should be done. At this time, one of the major short-term complications is infection.[13] Therefore, guidelines have to contain strict regulations as to which types of patients should receive ICDs. Overuse and misuse may be harmful for the whole ICD complex (and bad results can be the only gain from bad indications). Guidelines must set the path. Individual critical analysis of what is worth doing must be of concern for all those who are thinking of working with this fascinating technique.

The topic of guidelines is not new and the document shown in Figure 1 (see second paragraph, third column) explains the application of electricity to the chest for people who were supposed to be dead.

Participants of the Task Force of the Working Groups on Cardiac Arrhythmias and Cardiac Pacing of the European Society of Cardiology: G. Breithardt, A.J. Camm, R.W.F. Campbell, P. Coumel (Chairman), M.J. Janse, L. Kappenberger, H. Klein, K.H. Kuck, B. Lüderitz, N. Rehnqvist, P.J. Schwartz, P. Touboul. A Bayès de Luna, and H.J.J. Wellens (acting advisors). Writing Committee: A.J. Camm, R.W.F. Campbell, P. Coumel, M.J. Janse.

References

1. Lehmann MH, Saksena S: Implantable cardioverter defibrillators in cardiovascular practice: Report of the policy conference of the North American Society of Pacing and Electrophysiology. NASPE policy statement. PACE 1991; 14:969-979.
2. Steinbeck G, Meinertz T, Andresen D, et al: Empfehlungen zur Implantation von Defibrillatoren. Z Kardiol 1991; 80:475-478.
3. Crijns HJ, Hauer RNW, Kingma JH, et al: Cardiological Guidelines. Cardioverter defibrillator implantation. Neth J Cardiol 1991; 4:234-235.
4. Breithardt G, Camm AJ, Campbell RWF, et al: Guidelines for the use of implantable cardioverter defibrillators. A Task Force of the Working

Groups on Cardiac Arrhythmias and Cardiac Pacing of the European Society of Cardiology. Eur Heart J 1992; 13:1304-1310.
5. Bayès de Luna A, Coumel P, Leclercq JF: Ambulatory sudden cardiac death: Mechanisms of production of fatal arrhythmia on the basis of data from 157 cases. Am Heart J 1989; 117:151-159.
6. Kappenberger LJ, Del Bufalo A, Fromer MA: Termination and acceleration of ventricular tachycardia during antitachycardia pacing. In B Lüderitz, S Saksena (eds.): Interventional Electrophysiology. Mount Kisco, NY, Futura Publishing Co, 1991, pp. 225-231.
7. Fromer M, Schlaepfer J, Fischer A, et al: Experience with a new implantable pacer-cardioverter-defibrillator for the therapy of recurrent sustained ventricular tachyarrhythmias: A step toward a universal ventricular tachyarrhythmia control device. PACE 1991; 14:1288-1298.
8. Fromer M, Brachmann J, Block M, et al: Clinical experience with automatic electrical therapy for sustained ventricular tachycardia as delivered by a new implantable pacer-cardioverter defibrillator. Results of a European multicenter study incorporating 102 implants. Circulation 1992; 86:363-374.
9. Camilli L, Mugelli A, Grassi G, et al: Implantable pharmacological defibrillator: Preliminary investigations in animals. PACE 1991; 14:381-386.
10. Siebels J, Kuck KH: Effectiveness of antitachycardia pacing for ventricular tachycardia termination. In L Kappenberger, FW Lindemans (eds.): Practical Aspects of Staged Therapy Defibrillators. Mount Kisco, NY, Futura Publishing Co, 1992, pp. 39-42.
11. Lindemans FW, van Berlo AMW, Bourgeois IM: Summary of PCD™ clinical study results. In L Kappenberger, FW Lindemans (eds.): Practical Aspects of Staged Therapy Defibrillators. Mount Kisco, NY, Futura Publishing Co, 1992, pp. 103-111.
12. Saksena S, Tullo NG, Krol RB, et al: Initial clinical experience with endocardial defibrillation using an implantable cardioverter/defibrillator with a triple electrode system. Arch Intern Med 1989; 149:2333-2339.
13. Meesmann M: Factors associated with implantation-related complications. PACE 1992; 15:649-653.

7

Which Implantable Cardioverter-Defibrillator for which Patient?

Ph. Coumel

The implantable cardioverter-defibrillator (ICD) should not be considered only as a therapeutic tool. ICD technology offers a unique opportunity to extend our knowledge about infrequent, severe, or even lethal tachyarrhythmias. Unlike that from invasive electrophysiology, data provided by ICDs are limited to spontaneous phenomena. Therefore, the Holter philosophy and experience should be used to define pertinent data that should be sought for and stored. Three different categories relating to ICD technology can be distinguished, as described below.

1. Anecdotal data. Obtaining long electrocardiogram (ECG) strips immediately preceding the ICD intervention has an obvious interest. Such facilities are improving in the presently available devices and make them irreplaceable compared with conventional Holter. Although essential for documenting arrhythmias and checking the appropriateness of ICD interventions, such data have a limited value for understanding the phenomena since the important determinants may precede the intervention by minutes, hours, or days.

From *Transvenous Defibrillation and Radiofrequency Ablation* edited by A. John Camm and Fred W. Lindemans © 1995, Futura Publishing Co., Inc., Armonk, NY.

2. Storage algorithms. The presently limited ICD storage capacity necessitates careful decision of which data to store. Those dealing with the general outcome (arrhythmia quantification, cardiac frequency, sinus rate variability and, probably in the future, QT dynamicity) are identified but they can be monitored as well by conventional Holter. Those addressing the very tachyarrhythmias that form the targets for treatment (dependence on the prevailing rhythm and the autonomic nervous system, coupling intervals) are much less well-individualized and their relevance largely varies from patient to patient. Current storage limitations favor static rather than dynamic and much more informative time domain approaches. A comprehensive, comparative examination of the phenomena preceding specific arrhythmic events is needed, as individual cases hardly comply with standardized modes of computerized analysis.
3. Raw data storage. The main interest of ICD Holter over conventional Holter is to provide data concerning the real target arrhythmias rather than trivial surrogates, the significance and behavior of which may be inadequately extrapolated to critical events. Thus, the basic information formed by a time series of RR intervals and QRS types is the most important data, provided that they are stored in loops covering at least 24 hours, and that they are easily retrievable at any time for off-line analysis. Although at the present time such capabilities are limited by the available memory/energy in ICD technology, they form the essential first step for an improved knowledge and comprehension of the arrhythmias which the ICD is supposed to treat.

In conclusion, improving Holter facilities in the ICD is crucial for a better knowledge of tachyarrhythmias, a better management of patients and, thus, a better use of devices.

The ICD was developed as a therapeutic tool, although its potential diagnostic utilization was considered from the beginning by Mirowski.[1,2] Third generation devices that not only deliver high energy defibrillation shocks but also low energy cardioversion shocks and antitachycardia pacing fulfill the essential therapeutic needs. The technology has evolved from the original stages of spectacular lifesaving termination of lethal arrhythmias to more sophisticated and clinically transparent conversions of serious but not necessarily lethal tachyarrhythmias.

One can foresee that ICD therapeutic applications will not be limited to curative interventions. One can already think of preventive therapies using conventional pacing (prevention of pauses) or, more recently, subthreshold stimulation. However, any therapeutic progress is conditioned by an improvement in the knowledge that, in fact, may be a consequence of the therapeutic breakthrough itself. External defibrillation followed this process more than 25 years ago. What would be the current level of knowledge in clinical electrophysiology had the transthoracic defibrillation technique been confined to the intensive care unit without even recording the ECG? What would be the state of the art had resuscitation not been understood as giving the opportunity to safely investigate cardiac arrhythmias using provocative methods? Using the ICD to improve survival of patients with severe tachyarrhythmias is indeed important. Still, larger and larger series with prolonged follow-up show that, in the long term, an increase in cardiac deaths tends to compensate for a reduction in sudden death. As time elapses, the severity of the heart disease tends to make sudden death less "unexpected," as it is, after all, a modality of what is essentially cardiac death. There is a correlation between the difficulty of ICD indications and their benefits in terms of survival. It is rather easy statistically to evaluate the risk of sudden death in patients with a severely diseased heart, but the benefit of iterative resuscitations is not easy to evaluate.[3] On the other hand, the indication for an ICD may be much more difficult to decide in idiopathic ventricular fibrillation (VF), a poorly known entity,[4] but the benefit of successful resuscitation in this setting is unquestionable.

To further penetrate this difficult domain and, more generally, to improve our knowledge of spontaneous compared to artificially-induced tachyarrhythmias, collecting the information is essential. This aspect has been neglected in the first generations of ICDs for quite understandable technical reasons related to memory and energy limitations. Now that the longevity of the devices has substantially improved, the technical developments should be reoriented toward the collection of more information. Obviously, not all the patients have the same profile and need the same diagnostic and therapeutic approach. Thus, cardiologists have to think about what should be done technically to better meet the various needs of their patients.

Conventional Holter and Implanted Holter Functions

As a whole, the experience of conventional Holter should be referred to in order to define a strategy, keeping in mind the similarities and the differences between the external and implanted recording system. There are no memory or energy problems in the external Holter, at least if one does not consider the problems of digitizing an entire 24-hour, three-lead recording at a correct sampling rate and a good resolution,[5] a process that may require up to 300 MB of memory. Implanted Holter functions cannot yet play a role in this respect, partly because electrograms rather than ECGs are stored.

Conventional Holters are recorded with a circadian periodicity that looks quite natural. This is an important difference when compared to the implanted Holter, in which the time dimensions can be extended over weeks, months, or years. In conventional Holter, one is forced to record multiple tapes in order to be able to record rare events, and the quest for very rare events is hopeless. The opposite applies to the implanted Holter, which operates only when a therapeutic intervention is needed. Thus, schematically, the approach of recording frequent trivial events with one technique is in contrast with the approach of capturing exceptional events with the other. In the absence of any possible compromise, it has been considered in the past that a reliable image of the latter was yielded by the former. However, it has now been realized that such assumptions can be responsible for serious therapeutic mistakes.[6] In essence, the mistake came from the lack of information about really severe or even lethal tachyarrhythmias, so that life-threatening but fundamentally different arrhythmias were taken as surrogates. Severe tachyarrhythmias could only be artificially provoked so that the determinants of their spontaneous onset were necessarily unknown and, what is more serious, ignored. This is the reason why it came as a surprise to realize that drugs that were active on trivial arrhythmias could be inactive or even deleterious in other circumstances, whereas the contrary could apply to β-blockers.

One may distinguish three different levels of information in the data that may be obtained from ICD datalogs. For the time being, these levels are limited by technical considerations. However, the technical obstacles will be overcome, and the choice of which data are to be collected will be based on scientific consideration.

Anecdotal Data

To obtain traces as long as possible before the ICD intervention has an obvious interest. At first, only a few seconds of bipolar electrograms were available. The quality and duration of electrocardiographic tracings has now improved. Finally, one realizes that, in most cases, a simple marker of the ventricular activation is sufficient provided that it is highly reliable. The real interest of a digitized trace is to check the absence of artifacts, thus validating the appropriateness of the therapeutic intervention, the very reason for the recording itself.

The latter consideration actually forms the major limitation of these anecdotal data. They can only reflect the arrhythmic events for which the ICD has been programmed, not others. As a consequence, the information is limited to validating the normal functioning of the device or to detecting dysfunctions due to oversensing, not undersensing. In other words, the information is limited to the ICD itself and does not concern the heart and its arrhythmias. By definition, the long periods when the ICD made "no intervention" are not considered. At best, one may obtain fragments of data relating to aborted interventions (these are supposed to reflect self-limited arrhythmias) or unsuccessful attempts. This type of information is of course useful for tuning the parameters of ICD intervention or to evaluate the effects of medical therapy, but overall it is of limited importance.

Storage Algorithms

Limited storage capacity makes it necessary to strictly and parsimoniously define what data should be stored. Some types of information must not be expected from the ICD when they can easily be obtained from conventional Holter. This applies, for instance, to the quantification of trivial arrhythmias, the cardiac frequency or the heart rate variability, and probably, in the future, to QT dynamicity. Such parameters should not, however, be automatically discarded from the cadre of implanted Holter functions because they may acquire in this setting a renewed interest as the time dimension is extended over weeks, months, or years. Each of these parameters can be stored in the form of a single value obtained through relatively simple algorithms, the energy cost of which is limited. Spontaneous or drug-induced changes of heart rate variability or of QT dynamicity over long periods of time certainly will contribute important information for prognosis as well as for the therapeutic effects.

In fact, one mainly expects from implanted Holter to obtain more complete information on rare events that are not recorded by conventional Holter. The impossibility of storing everything over prolonged periods makes it necessary to define storage algorithms in the same way as intervention algorithms. This requires making predefined choices concerning the events that will be considered in order to precisely define their nature, to classify and to date them, and to look for their determinants. At each and every step, one is at risk of making wrong choices because, in essence, one has to define what is being looked for without having the possibility to validate the choices, the risk being to ignore the really important information.

One can easily find an example of such difficulties in the domain of sudden death recorded on Holter tapes. The reported cases[7] show how meticulous the analysis should be. Considering only primary VF, it is now established that it is often preceded by a progressive acceleration of heart rate over several minutes or tens of minutes, thus suggesting the existence of adrenergic stimulation as a causal factor. On the other hand, torsades de pointes, another arrhythmia responsible for sudden death, is usually preceded by a trend of heart rate decrease. If these two opposite behaviors are mixed by not differentiating primary VF from torsades de pointes, the correct information would be missed in both cases. Such a situation is indeed observed in the literature and will necessarily occur with storage algorithms that cannot achieve this somewhat difficult electrocardiographic diagnosis.

The present memory limitations favor "static" storage algorithms in the form of RR interval histograms, of which the number and capacity can be multiplied at a low cost in terms of energy and memory. The interest of such an approach is limited because it neglects the importance of considering sequences of cycles rather than cycle intervals as such. Still, some relatively simple arrhythmias can be quantified, and this representation gives a very global and approximative image of heart variability.

Dynamic algorithms are more informative as they allow display of the trends of rate that may precede the arrhythmic events. The upper panel of Figure 1 clearly shows the trend of heart rate slowing that precedes an isolated premature beat and then the tachycardia onset just after the pause. The lower panel illustrates the therapeutic impact such information may have if an adequate postextrasystolic stimulation can intervene to prevent the tachycardia. Such information is important when one knows that about 50% of recorded sudden death episodes show the presence of a pause as one of the determinants of the arrhythmic event.[7]

One can imagine a number of storage algorithms that have in common saving energy and memory. However, they also have in common targeting this or that type of event, and ignoring what is not targeted. In ICD patients, the philosophy must be that the targets are by definition rare. To evaluate their exact significance implies that they should be compared to much more trivial events in order to define the relevant determinants. But these trivial events themselves must be

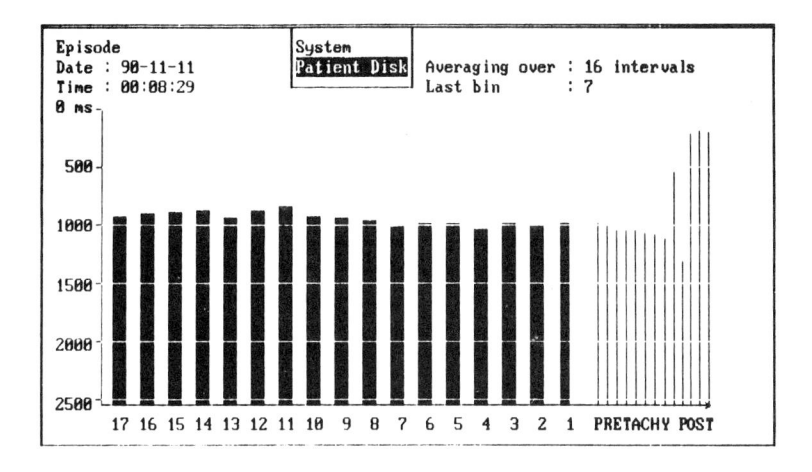

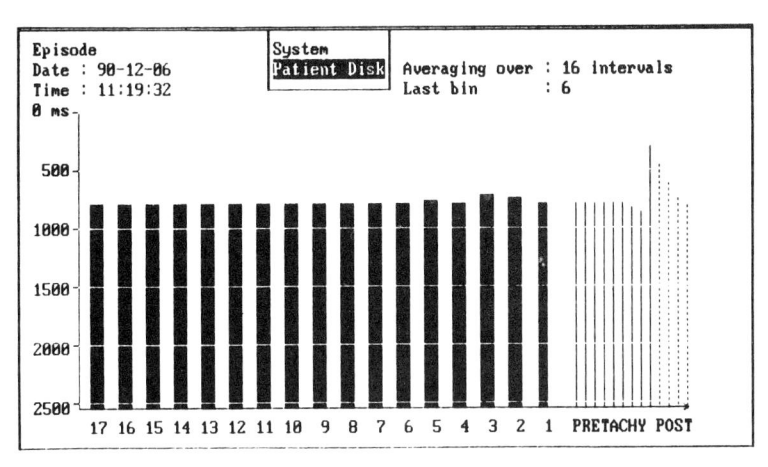

Figure 1. *In this prototype pacemaker (Medtronic Prometheus™), the onset of the tachyarrhythmias can be detected and stored on a beat-by-beat basis for the first beats of the arrhythmia and the last preceding sinus cycles. During the five previous minutes, the cardiac cycles are averaged and displayed as bins of 16 intervals. The upper panel shows the mode of onset of the tachyarrhythmia: an isolated premature beat is preceded by a progressive slowing of the sinus rhythm, and the pause secondary to this extrasystole apparently triggers the arrhythmia. The lower panel shows how a therapeutic consequence can be drawn from this information, in the form of a rate-smoothing stimulation that is triggered by the initial premature beat. Please note the reversed interval scale on the vertical axis. Paced intervals in the lower panel are represented by dotted lines.*

compared to something else, and the notion of attempting to record the absence of an event is difficult. It implies that there is a need for recording long and more complete information.

One may conclude that storage algorithms have that particular interest to obviate some of the present limitations of ICD technology. They are, however, far from providing a solution for all problems. Still, they can help to solve the well-identified problems, once the right way of quantification is determined.

Raw Data Storage

The main interest of implanted Holter compared to conventional Holter is to provide data concerning the arrhythmias that form the real targets for treatment, rather than the surrogates. The basic information routinely used by the cardiologist is the ECG. Technically speaking, this is the most difficult challenge for collection and storage. Fortunately, it is not necessary to have the complete information all the time, so that it can be usefully analyzed prior to storage. The sequence of RR intervals and the indication of normal or abnormal patterns of QRS complexes already contain the main information on arrhythmias, cardiac frequency, and heart rate variability. In the future, they will probably be combined with information on the ST-T segment and the QT interval.

To exploit this information that is presented as a 24-hour loop is the ideal way of using the possibilities of implanted Holter functions. The fact that it cannot yet be a reality must not prevent this being considered as an important objective. As a matter of fact, the improved knowledge it will provide will be crucial for the improving the management of the arrhythmias with which the ICD is expected to deal with.

Off-line processing of these raw data is the only way to have full flexibility and to develop new algorithms for exploiting new data. What is expected from the Holter technology is to provide easy access to hitherto rare exceptional data as soon as they are collected and as often as necessary. In this domain, transtelephonic transmission will be extremely useful not only to make the data quickly available but also to save them. With this philosophy, we can renew the approach of clinical electrophysiology to the same extent as what was done in the past with provocative methods.

Conclusion

One must be conscious that many essential technical improvements cannot be achieved as yet. In addition, not all of them are necessary in all patients. Some patients, whose problems are fully identified, only need the full therapeutic capacity of the device. In contrast, other patients have a low probability of ICD interventions, but there may exist a crucial need for data about their arrhythmias and the causative disease. One may conceive that various ICD models can be tailored to meet the particular problems of each patient. The ideal device should have a full versatility between the therapeutic and the diagnostic functions.

References

1. Mirowski M, Mower MM: The automatic implantable defibrillator: Some historical notes. In P Brugada, HJJ Wellens (eds.): Cardiac Arrhythmias: Where to Go from Here? Mount Kisco, NY, Futura Publishing Co Inc, 1987, pp. 655-662.
2. Coumel P: Historical milestones of implanted defibrillators. PACE 1992; 15(III):598-603.
3. Task Force of the Working Group on Cardiac Arrhythmias and Cardiac Pacing of the European Society of Cardiology: Guidelines for the use of implantable cardioverter defibrillators. Eur Heart J 1992; 13:1304-1310.
4. Priori SG, Borggrefe M, Camm AJ, et al: Unexplained cardiac arrest. The need for a prospective registry. Eur Heart J 1992; 13:1445-1446. Editorial.
5. Coumel Ph, Maison-Blanche P: Electrocardiography and computers. J Amb Monit 1992; 5:265-272.
6. Akhtar M, Breithardt G, Camm AJ, et al: Implications of the cardiac arrhythmia suppression trial. Eur Heart J 1990; 11:194-199.
7. Leclercq JF, Maison-Blanche P, Cauchemez B, et al: Respective role of sympathetic tone and of cardiac pauses in the genesis of 62 cases of ventricular fibrillation recorded during Holter monitoring. Eur Heart J 1988; 9:1276-1283.

8

Surgical Aspects of Cardioverter-Defibrillator Implantation

F. Veit

Several techniques exist for implanting cardioverter-defibrillators, but they all have the same objectives: to establish adequate electrogram sensing and arrhythmia detection, to provide effective and reliable arrhythmia termination, and to limit the incidence of acute and chronic surgical complications. The surgical approaches for positioning the defibrillation electrodes include median sternotomy, distal median sternotomy, left (antero) lateral thoracotomy, subxyphoidal access to the heart, the subcostal approach, and the nonthoracotomy, endocardial implantation technique, with or without a subcutaneous patch electrode. This last approach has become the method of choice in most centers.

Advantages of the median sternotomy for placing epicardial electrodes are that this approach allows combined procedures and provides excellent exposure. Patches can be precisely positioned and affixed to the epicardium or the pericardium, pace-sense electrodes can be placed in an optimal position along the obtuse margin of the left ventricle, various patch positions can be tested to obtain a low defibrillation threshold (DFT), and it is possible to also use the procedure after previous cardiac surgery.

From *Transvenous Defibrillation and Radiofrequency Ablation* edited by A. John Camm and Fred W. Lindemans © 1995, Futura Publishing Co., Inc., Armonk, NY.

Disadvantages of the median sternotomy are the potential for sternal infection (0.5% to 1.5%), the incidence of atelectasis, and the need for respiratory support. The procedure may cause pericardial effusion, possibly requiring pericardial drainage. The patient must, at least temporarily, be admitted to the surgical intensive care unit and pneumothorax may develop. All these disadvantages are characteristic for cardiac surgery.

Advantages of the left thoracotomy as an approach for defibrillator implantation are that it provides good exposure, it allows epicardial as well as pericardial patch fixation, and it provides an option for combined transvenous/patch implants as well as for patch/patch lead configurations.

Disadvantages are that the patient often suffers more pain after the procedure, that atelectasis may occur, and that thoracotomy drainage is required. Also, DFTs are reported to be 15% to 20% higher than when electrodes are placed via the sternotomy approach.

Advantages of the subcostal approach, as developed by Lawrie et al,[1] are that opening of the pleural cavity is not necessary, thereby avoiding pleural effusions, that access to the left ventricle is good, that atelectasis will not occur, and that postsurgical pain is minimal. Extubation can take place immediately after the implant procedure and the patient can be mobilized soon after the operation, leading to a short hospital stay. The procedure allows the use of the spring/patch electrode configuration and there is no need for lead tunnelling or more than one incision.

Disadvantages of the subcostal approach are that a mini-thoracotomy may be required in about 13% of patients and that positioning of pace-sense screw-in leads may be difficult.

The advantages of the subxiphoid approach, as described by Watkins et al,[2] are that there is no need for opening the pleural cavity, thereby avoiding the risk of pleural effusions or atelectasis and that postsurgical pain is minimal. Immediate extubation and early mobilization lead to a short hospital stay and patch/patch as well as spring/patch electrode configurations are possible.

Disadvantages of this procedure are that it is not possible after previous cardiac surgery and that positioning of two patches and of the pace-sense electrodes may be difficult due to the limited exposure.

Implantation of a cardioverter defibrillator requires general anesthesia with intubation, possibly single lung ventilation in case of a left thoracotomy; a multi-channel electrocardiogram recorder; an intraarterial pressure line, optionally a Swan-Ganz catheter; a Foley catheter; an external rescue defibrillator with stick-on chest electrodes or (sterile) chest paddles (sterile cardiac paddles for epicardial patch implants); an introducer set for subclavian vein puncture; C-arm fluoroscopy; and the perioperative administration of antibiotics, which we give in a monotherapy mode for at least three to four days. In addition, equipment is needed to test DFTs, electrogram amplitudes, and pacing thresholds of the implanted leads and to induce ventricular fibrillation.

The nonthoracotomy approach, with which we now have experience in 54 patients, is clearly the least invasive method to implant a defibrillator. Lead insertion requires slight elevation of the left thorax, facilitating a pocket formation for the subcutaneous electrode, and a moderate Trendelenburg's position. After a small skin incision, access to the venous system can be obtained through the cephalic vein and/ or through the subclavian vein by means of subclavian puncture using an introducer set.

Although two leads can be entered into the subclavian vein through either double puncture or through the double guide-wire method, it is strongly recommended to use the cephalic route for the ventricular lead that, due to its larger diameter and multi-conductor construction, is most vulnerable for being damaged when compressed in the area between the clavicle and the first rib. Access to a small cephalic vein can be facilitated with an introducer and it is essential to use a lateral site of entry when an introducer is used for the subclavian vein.

It is equally important to carefully secure the leads using the anchoring sleeves and to form a loop in the lead body close to the entry site for preventing lead migration. The suture that fixates the lead inside the anchoring sleeve should not be used at the same time to fix the anchoring sleeve to the tissue because subsequent tissue necrosis within the suture may make it loose. Absorbable suture material must never be used for lead fixation.

Figure 1 illustrates what careful fixation of the anchoring sleeves and formation of a loop in the electrode body will prevent: dislocation of the superior vena cava (SVC) lead.

The preferred method of implanting the implantable cardioverter-defibrillator (ICD) device itself is in the upper left quadrant of the abdomen behind the rectus muscle. Instead of a transverse incision of the muscle, we prefer a longitudinal incision, which makes it easy to proceed with a subxyphoid implant approach in case the nonthoracotomy implantation fails.

Possible surgery-related complications are lead migration; patch crinkling; damage to lead insulation; perforation of the right ventricle; lead conductor fracture; infection of the generator pocket, of the subcu-

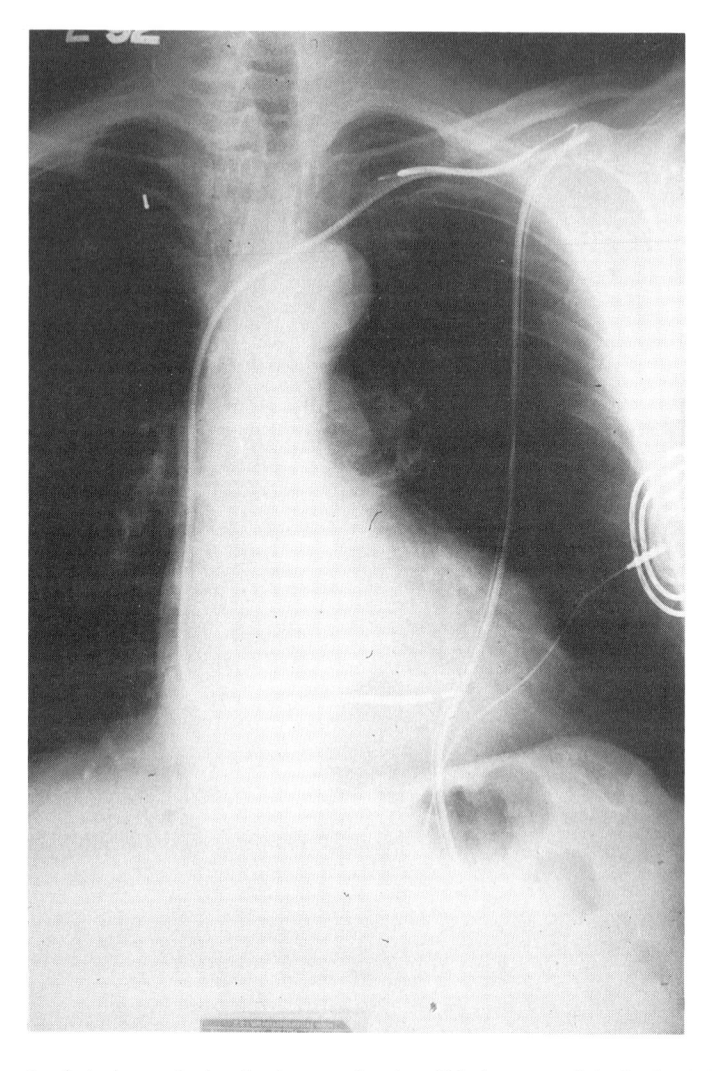

86 • TRANSVENOUS DEFIBRILLATION AND RF ABLATION

Figure 1. *Anterior-posterior chest x-ray showing dislodgement of the lead originally positioned in the SVC.*

taneous lead pocket, of the venous access site, or possibly of the whole system; thrombosis; perforation or erosion of the generator pocket; and seroma or hematoma in the pocket of the device or of the subcutaneous patch electrode. Implantation of epicardial patch electrodes carries the risks of the procedure used to obtain access to the heart as well as the patch-specific risks of bleeding from coronary arteries or veins, (constrictive) pericarditis, and laceration of the ascending aorta if patches are positioned too high.

Between May, 1989 and February, 1993, the First and the Fourth Surgical Departments of the Vienna-Lainz University Hospital and the Third Medical Department of the Vienna Wilhelminen Hospital implanted 76 defibrillators. Sternotomy was applied in 22 patients. Fifty-four patients implanted during the last two years received the defibrillator via the nonthoracotomy approach. Of the 22 patients undergoing sternotomy, 7 received coronary artery bypass grafts and 1 of these patients also received a mitral valve during the ICD implant procedure.

An attempt to implant a transvenous/subcutaneous lead system in 54 patients was made. Using 24 J as the maximum acceptable DFT, the primary success rate was 94.5%: 51 patients met the DFT criterion and received the intended lead system. In two patients, a subxyphoid approach had to be used and the procedure was aborted in one patient until a device with biphasic output would be available.

Variations of lead configuration or switching between sequential and simultaneous current delivery modes were necessary in 4 of the 54 patients in order to obtain success with the nonthoracotomy approach.

Perioperative complications of all 76 patients who received an ICD can be summarized as follows:

Sternotomy group: 22 patients:

- two patients died, one due to a myocardial infarction and one due to a cerebrovascular accident and
- no patients suffered an infection during the perioperative phase.

Nonsternotomy group: 54 patients:

- no patients died perioperatively;
- no patients suffered an infection during the perioperative phase;
- two patients experienced a hematoma in the subcutaneous patch pocket and one of them was under heparin treatment because of previous mitral valve replacement;
- two patients experienced a pneumothorax; and
- one patient had a DFT >34 J (implantation was postponed until a device with biphasic output would be available) and two other patients had high DFTs and underwent subxyphoidal procedures.

Late complications requiring reoperation in the 74 patients who had received an ICD and were discharged from the hospital were observed as follows during an average follow-up of 14 months, ranging from 1 to 44 months:

- six patients had problems with the generator pocket: perforation or erosion occurred in three patients, two of whom had the device implanted subcutaneously, and the device displaced to a subcostal position in one patient and connector problems required reoperation in two patients;
- three patients experienced dislodgement of the SVC lead during the second postimplant month and in one of them the right ventricular lead dislodged as well;
- one patient suffered thrombosis in the SVC; and
- five patients experienced problems with the subcutaneous patch electrode between 2 and 32 months postimplant: crinkling and substantial fibrosis were observed in four patients and erosion and bleeding were observed in one patient.

Overall, reoperation for late complications was required in 14 patients. This late complication rate of 18.5% should drop substantially when pocket problems can be avoided through smaller devices and submuscular implantation, when lead dislodgement is prevented through improved anchoring techniques, and when the use of the subcutaneous patch electrode can be avoided through lower DFTs in devices with biphasic output.

Figure 2 shows an x-ray of a patient experiencing substantial crinkling of the subcutaneous patch electrode, combined with excessive fibrosis, 32 months after implantation.

Conclusions

Our data indicate that nonthoracotomy lead systems can be implanted safely with monophasic or biphasic defibrillators and that acceptable DFTs can be obtained in about 95% of patients. This makes their use the approach of first choice in patients requiring ICD therapy.

The subxyphoid or subcostal approach is the second method of choice in patients without previous sternotomy (cardiac surgery) if DFTs are too high even with the use of a biphasic defibrillation pulse.

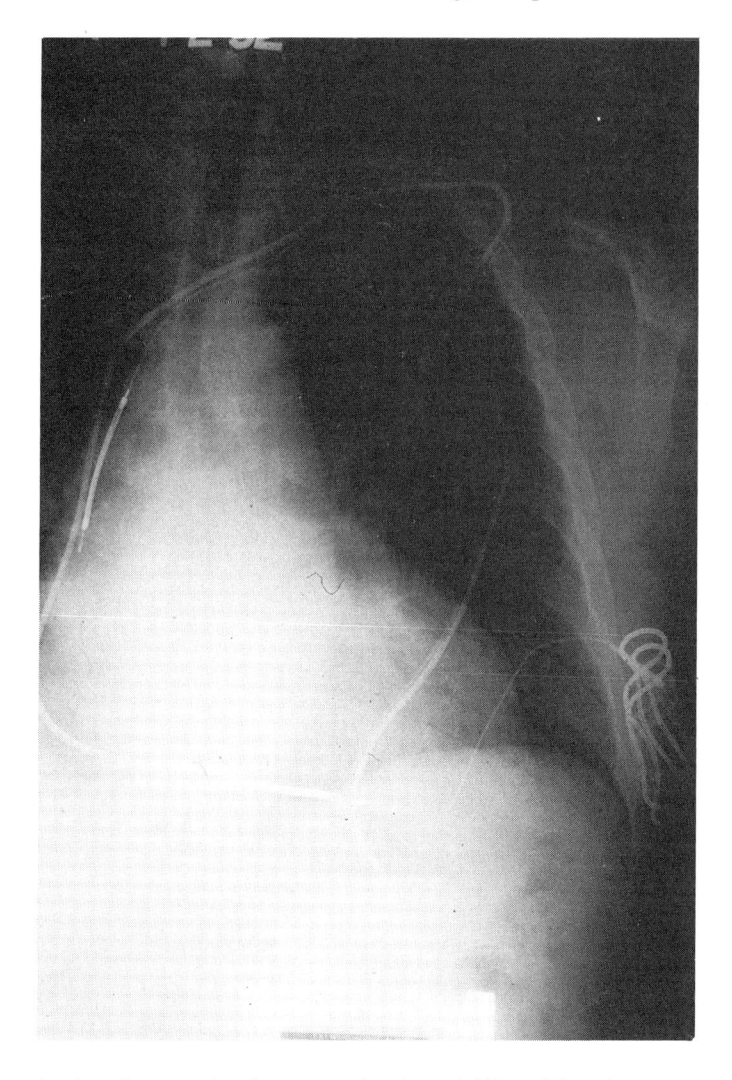

Figure 2. *Anterior-posterior chest x-ray showing crinkling of the subcutaneous patch electrode.*

If the implantation of a nonthoracotomy lead system fails to provide adequate DFTs, an anterolateral thoracotomy is the procedure of choice in patients with previous cardiac surgery.

Placement of the defibrillator device in a position behind the rectus abdominis muscle generally avoids reoperations for complications related to the generator pocket. Lead migration should be avoided by implanting the lead with a loop in the area of venous access, by using the anchoring sleeves for the lead, and by verifying their hold on the lead. Problems related to the subcutaneous patch will probably be reduced when defibrillators with biphasic output reduce the need for their use.

References

1. Lawrie GM, Griffin J, Wyndham C: Epicardial implantation of automatic implantable defibrillator by left subcostal thoracotomy. PACE 1984; 7:1370.
2. Watkins L, Mirowski M, Mower MM, et al: Implantation of the automatic defibrillator: The subxiphoid approach. Ann Thorac Surg 1982; 34:515.

9

Influence of Electrode Position on Defibrillation Threshold

J. Winter, C. Perings, T. Cappel, S. Kuhls, M. Pauschinger, E.G. Vester, H.D. Schulte

Apart from the shock waveform, the current pathway and the amount of energy delivered by an implantable cardioverter-defibrillator and the electrode size and placement influence the success rate of defibrillation shocks. Animal studies and clinical investigations showed that defibrillation threshold (DFT) decreased as the surface area increased up to a critical patch size.[1,2]

The mean DFTs of a two-patch lead system were typically around 10 J and remained stable over time in the majority of the patients.[3] In view of the comparatively small surface area of the so-called "nonthoracotomy" leads (Table 1), it has generally been recommended that an additional subcutaneous/submuscular patch electrode be implanted in order to ensure adequate magnitude of the cardioverting electrical field.[4] Early trials suggested that an accessory patch electrode was always necessary to achieve DFTs at or below 20 J.[5-10]

The effects of electrode position on DFTs have not been investigated extensively. Our own and other studies have shown that dual epicardial electrode systems should encompass as much ventricular mass as possible.[11] It is recommended that one patch should be placed

From *Transvenous Defibrillation and Radiofrequency Ablation* edited by A. John Camm and Fred W. Lindemans © 1995, Futura Publishing Co., Inc., Armonk, NY.

Table 1
Electrode Surface Areas

Vena cava + epicardial patch lead system	≈ 3460 mm^2
Double patch lead system	≈ 5600 mm^2
Intracardial lead system + SQ-patch	≈ 3790 mm^2
Intracardial lead system	≈ 990 mm^2

on the left ventricle and another placed as diametrically opposite as possible on the right ventricle. Final acceptance of epicardial electrode positions must depend on the result of DFT testing.

There are three locations for placing the endocardial lead electrodes: superior vena cava (SVC)/right atrium, coronary sinus, and right ventricle. The easiest method of endocardial defibrillation is to deliver a shock between two electrodes in the right side of the heart, usually placed in the right ventricular apex and the right atrium/SVC junction. Experimental and human studies have shown that this technique is successful despite the lack of an electrode near to the left ventricle.[12-14] An improved current distribution is achieved when a patch electrode is implanted subcutaneously. The advantage of a coronary sinus lead in combination with a right ventricular lead consists in application of a higher transmyocardial voltage gradient to the lateral and basal left ventricle. Despite these theoretical advantages, two clinical studies using totally endocardial lead systems including the coronary sinus failed to show a success rate exceeding 50% at an energy level of 18 J or less.[15,16] Furthermore, it is not always possible to cannulate the coronary sinus, and lead dislodgement from a coronary sinus position is a frequently reported complication.[17]

Study Objective

The goal of our study was to investigate the possibility of obtaining DFTs of 15 J or less with a single endocardial lead in absence of a subcutaneous patch electrode. The distal coil of the electrode should be positioned against the endocardium of the septum to improve the current density to this part of the left ventricle. If a DFT of >15 J should be achieved, the lead had to be repositioned despite sufficient pacing parameters.

Methods

Study Patients

Thirty-eight consecutive patients requiring a cardioverter-defibrillator for recurrent sustained ventricular tachycardia (17 patients) and/or aborted sudden cardiac death (21 patients) were investigated for single endocardial lead implantation. The mean age (±standard deviation) of 11 female and 27 male patients was 59±11.2 years. Coronary artery heart disease was present in 26 cases. Five patients suffered from nonischemic dilative cardiomyopathy, and two suffered from hypertrophic obstructive cardiomyopathy. In four patients, primary electrical disease was suggested. One patient suffered from long QT syndrome.

Thirteen patients underwent previous cardiac surgery. Three of these patients had been operated on twice before. Each patient underwent cardiac catheterization with angiography and baseline electrophysiological study. The mean left ventricular ejection fraction was 41.7±14.9%, with a range from 14% to 77%.

Intraoperative Procedure

In all cases, we used a 12 F single tripolar, endocardial cardioversion/defibrillation and pacing lead. In 95% of all patients, venous access was obtained via the cephalic vein through a small incision in the deltopectoral groove. Correct positioning of the distal coil of the lead next to the septum was the vital factor in the success that has been achieved using this implantation technique. The proximal electrode was positioned in the SVC/right atrium junction (Fig. 1). When the lead was placed in a supposedly optimal position, sensing and pacing parameter measurements were performed with a pacing system analyzer.

Our study protocol required pacing thresholds of <1.0 V at 0.5 millisecond pulse duration and electrogram amplitude and slew rate >5.0 mV and 0.5 V/second, respectively, in sinus rhythm. If pacing parameters fell outside these ranges, the endocardial lead was repositioned. Contrary to some isolated reports, repositioning is perfectly feasible. The stylet is advanced to the lead tip and the lead is withdrawn 1 to 2 cm and then repositioned. Morphology sensing amplitude was measured from a multi-channel strip chart recorder connected to an external cardioverter-defibrillator. A morphology sensing amplitude of ≥3 mV was accepted.

94 • TRANSVENOUS DEFIBRILLATION AND RF ABLATION

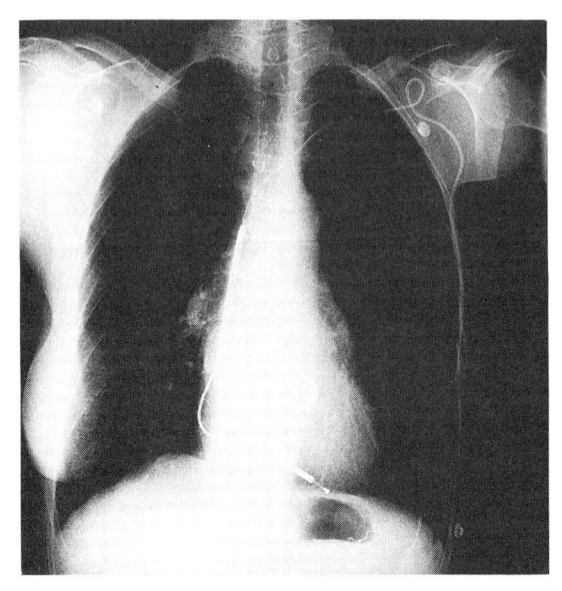

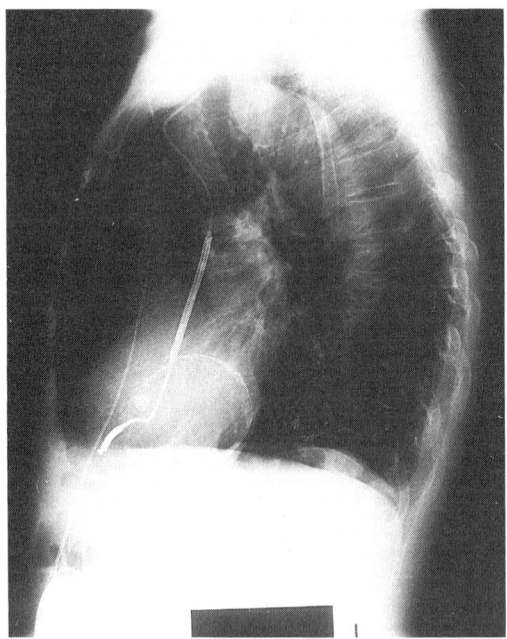

Figure 1. *Anteroposterior (upper) and lateral (lower) x-rays showing correct position of the distal coil next to the ventricular septum. The obtained DFT was 8 J using monophasic shock waveform.*

Defibrillation threshold was then determined, following alternating current-induced ventricular fibrillation (VF), the first shock being 15 J. In case of defibrillation, subsequent shocks in sequence of 10, 8, and 5 J were applied. Five minutes elapsed between every VF episode. The criterion for implantation of the single endocardial lead was three successful conversions of VF using 15 J or less. In the current series of 38 patients, after lead repositioning, four of the five patients showed an improved DFT. If the minimum achievable DFT was greater than 15 J despite repositioning, a subcutaneous electrode was inserted. Wherever possible, biphasic shocks were used as they permit lower thresholds with a greater margin of safety.

Intraoperative Results

Pacing parameters were sufficient in 35 patients for the first lead position. In 33 of the 38 patients, induced VF was successfully terminated at 20 J or less (Table 2). In one patient with a DFT of 20 J, a subcutaneous patch electrode was implanted without reduction of the DFT. In this case, it was not attempted to reposition the endocardial lead. Repositioning of the endocardial electrode was necessary in five cases in which DFTs were above 20 J. In one patient, repositioning was immediately successful, and in the other two cases, two attempts were necessary to achieve a DFT of 15 J or less. Despite multiple repositioning of the endocardial lead in two patients, the obtained DFTs were 20 and 40 J, respectively. In these two cases, a subcutaneous patch electrode was implanted. In one case, the DFT decreased from 20 to 10 J, while in the second patient, the DFT remained at 40 J. In 35 cases, termination of induced VF using a 15 J monophasic or biphasic shock waveform or less was possible.

In 15 cases, devices delivering biphasic shock waveforms were available. The DFTs achieved by monophasic shock waveforms were

Table 2
Intraoperative Results

	DFT ≤15 J	DFT 20 J	DFT >20 J
1 electrode position	32	1*	5
2 electrode positions	1	—	—
>2 electrode positions	2	1	1

DFT: defibrillation threshold; *: no repositioning of the lead; a subcutaneous patch was implanted without reduction of the defibrillation threshold.

compared with those achieved by biphasic shock waveforms in only the first seven cases. In these cases, the DFT was significantly lower for the biphasic pulses. Thirty-five out of 38 patients met our implant criterion for single endocardial lead implantation. The mean DFT of all implanted patients was 10.4±4.0 J. The DFT achieved by monophasic shock waveforms was 11.9±3.6 J, with biphasic shock waveform respectively 8±2.9 J.

Postoperative Course

There were no intraoperative or perioperative surgery complications. Prior to discharge, VF was induced in all patients and effectively terminated by the first shock with a safety margin of 10 J above the intraoperatively determined DFT.

Seventeen patients with a minimum follow-up of two months were reassessed. In 13 of the 17 patients, termination of induced VF was achieved with the same minimal energy requirement as obtained intraoperatively. In one patient, the DFT increased by 5 J, and in two patients, the DFT increased by 10 J. In another patient, x-ray revealed dislocation of the endocardial lead. The cardioverter-defibrillator failed to defibrillate induced VF within the 30 J energy level in this patient. Pacing and sensing parameters were sufficient at reoperation. Attempts to remove the endocardial lead were unsuccessful and a submuscular patch electrode was implanted. The DFT was 10 J.

Conclusion

Effective defibrillation within a 15 J energy level is possible in nearly all cases using an endocardial lead system.

Energy requirements depend on lead position. Successful positioning of the distal right ventricular electrode against the endocardium of the intraventricular septum is the key factor in the success of our technique since it allows maximal contact and thereby substantially reduces DFTs. This is especially illustrated by a patient with a left ventricular ejection fraction of 14% in whom a DFT of 5 J, using a monophasic shock waveform, was obtained.

As indicated, lead repositioning is both feasible and practicable when required. In the current series of 38 patients, four of the five patients with an initially high DFT had their lead repositioned which resulted in an improved DFT.

Despite stable DFTs in most of our patients, an energy safety margin of about 15 J between acute DFT and cardioverter-defibrillator energy rating is currently desirable to ensure successful postoperative defibrillation. Routine x-rays and electrophysiological studies are necessary to detect asymptomatic lead dislodgement and to explain a possible rise of DFT.

In our experience, the simplest method of defibrillation achieved by an entirely endocardial lead system will soon be the gold standard.

References

1. Dixon EG, Tang AS, Wolf PD, et al: Improved defibrillation thresholds with large contoured epicardial electrodes and biphasic waveforms. Circulation 1987; 76:1176-1181.
2. Mehra R, DeGroot PJ, Norenberg MS: Energy waveforms and lead systems for implantable defibrillators. In B Lüderitz, S Saksena (eds.): Interventional Electrophysiology. Mount Kisco, NY, Futura Publishing Co, 1991, pp. 377-394.
3. Wetherbee JN, Chapmann PD, Troup PJ, et al: Long-term internal cardiac defibrillation threshold stability. PACE 1989; 12:443-449.
4. Wetherbee JN, Chapmann PD, Klopfenstein HS, et al: Nonthoracotomy internal defibrillation in dogs: Threshold reduction using a subcutaneous chest wall electrode with a transvenous catheter electrode. J Am Coll Cardiol 1987; 10:406-411.
5. Winkle RA, Bach SM, Mead RH, et al: Comparison of defibrillation efficacy in humans using a new catheter and superior vena cava spring-left ventricular patch electrodes. J Am Coll Cardiol 1988; 11:365-370.
6. Saksena S, Parsonnet V: Implantation of cardioverter/defibrillator without thoracotomy using a triple electrode system. JAMA 1988; 259:69-72.
7. Saksena S, Tullo NG, Krol RB, et al: Initial clinical experience with endocardial defibrillation using an implantable cardioverter/defibrillator with a triple-electrode system. Arch Intern Med 1989; 149:2333-2339.
8. McCowan R, Maloney J, Wilkoff B, et al: Automatic implantable cardioverter-defibrillator implantation without thoracotomy using an endocardial and submuscular patch system. J Am Coll Cardiol 1991; 17:415-421.
9. Moore SL, Maloney JD, Edel TB, et al: Implantable cardioverter defibrillator implanted by nonthoracotomy approach: Initial clinical experience with the redesigned transvenous lead system. PACE 1991; 14:1865-1869.
10. Saksena S, Mehta D, Krol RB, et al: Experience with a third-generation implantable cardioverter-defibrillator. Am J Cardiol 1991; 67:1375-1384.
11. Hopps JA, Bigelow WG: Electrical treatment of cardiac arrest: A cardiac stimulator/defibrillator. Surgery 1954; 36:833-849.
12. Mirowski M, Mower MM, Staewen WS, et al: Standby automatic defibrillator. An approach to prevention of sudden coronary death. Arch Intern Med 1970; 126:158-161.
13. Mirowski M, Mower MM, Gott VL, et al: Feasibility and effectiveness of low-energy catheter defibrillation in man. Circulation 1973; 47:79-85.

14. Winter J, Vester EG, Kuhls S, et al: Defibrillation energy requirements with single endocardial (Endotak™) lead. PACE 1993; 16:540-546.
15. Bardy GH, Allen MD, Mehra R: Transvenous defibrillation in humans via the coronary sinus. Circulation 1990; 81:1252-1259.
16. Yee R, Klein GJ, Leitch JW, et al: A permanent transvenous lead system for an implantable pacemaker cardioverter/defibrillator. Circulation 1992; 85:196-204.
17. European PCD™ Study. Patients with Transvene™ Lead Systems. Clinical Evaluation Report. Medtronic Bakken Research Center, Maastricht, The Netherlands, 1991.

10

Implantable Transvenous Cardioverter-Defibrillator with Pectoral Subcutaneous Patch

S. Favale, M.V. Pitzalis, G. Luzzi,
C.D. Dicandia, C. Forleo, G. Mannatrizio,
P. Tunzi, M. Di Biase, P. Rizzon

More effective lead systems and biphasic defibrillation waveforms have facilitated transvenous implantation. Biomedical advances leading to smaller defibrillators will make pectoral implantation the procedure of choice, especially in combination with the active defibrillator can serving as one of the electrodes.[1] Some experimental procedures have already demonstrated the possibility of cardioverter-defibrillator implantation with transvenous leads in combination with the subcutaneous patch in the pectoral position.[2,3]

The aim of this study was to evaluate a new technique for implanting a pectoral subcutaneous patch electrode that reduces the number of incisions from three to two.

Method

Since June, 1992, a modified cardioverter-defibrillator implant technique has been evaluated in seven consecutive patients. Clinical data of

From *Transvenous Defibrillation and Radiofrequency Ablation* edited by A. John Camm and Fred W. Lindemans © 1995, Futura Publishing Co., Inc., Armonk, NY.

the patient population are summarized in Table 1. An incision along the left deltopectoral groove or in the left subclavicular region (Fig. 1) was made for inserting both the right ventricular (RV, Medtronic 6966) and the superior vena cava (SVC, Medtronic 6963) catheters through the left cephalic and/or subclavian vein and for placing the chest patch in a subcutaneous intraclavicular pocket (Medtronic 6999–6921).

Defibrillation testing began by examining defibrillation efficacy of a 24 J sequential pulse using the RV electrode as the common cathode, the high superior vena cava- (SVC-) left brachiocephalic vein electrode as the pulse-1 anode, and the pectoral patch as the pulse-2 anode (Fig. 2).

If defibrillation was unsuccessful with the sequential pulse method at 24 J, a rescue pulse was delivered and testing was repeated 4 minutes

Table 1
Description of the Patient Population

Clinical Data

Patient	Age	Gender	LVEF	Arrhythmia	Disease
1	65	M	17%	VT	CAD
2	67	M	45%	VT	CAD
3	70	M	46%	VT	DCM
4	66	M	26%	VT/VF	CAD
5	46	M	30%	VT/VF	CHD
6	60	M	28%	VT/VF	CAD
7	69	M	46%	VT	CAD

VT: ventricular tachycardia; VF: ventricular fibrillation; CAD: coronary artery disease; CHD: congenital heart disease; DCM: dilated cardiomyopathy; LVEF: left ventricular ejection fraction

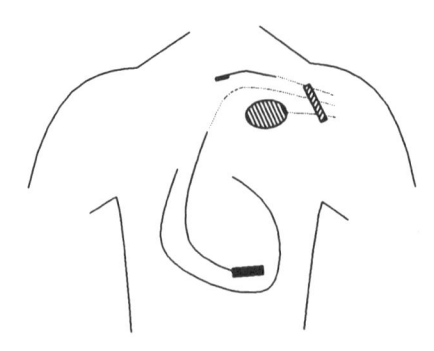

Figure 1. *Right ventricular lead, SVC or left brachiocephalic lead, and patch lead are all inserted via one incision.*

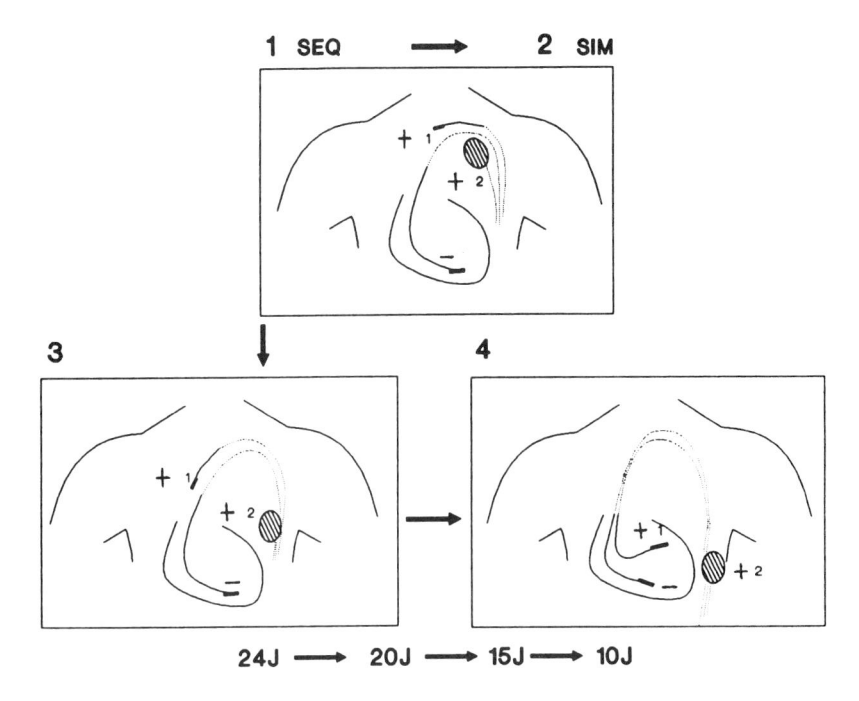

Figure 2. *Schematic representation of the sequence of lead configuration and DFT testing. See text for explanation.*

later using a 24 J simultaneous pulse with the same electrode configuration and polarity. If 24 J simultaneous pulsing failed, the more common configuration using the SVC electrode in a lower position and a self-adhesive cutaneous patch in the axillary or apical position was tested. The following step, if necessary, included the use of the coronary sinus and the implantation of an extrapericardial patch (hybrid configuration).

The implantation criterion required three out of four consecutive successful terminations of ventricular fibrillation (VF) with an output energy of 24 J or less. In four of the five patients in whom, when using the pectoral patch, defibrillation was successful at 24 J, defibrillation threshold (DFT) was measured by decremental energy testing (24 to 20 to 15 to 10 J).

Results

Five of the 7 patients were implanted with a subcutaneous patch in the pectoral position (Fig. 3 and Table 2). In the four patients in

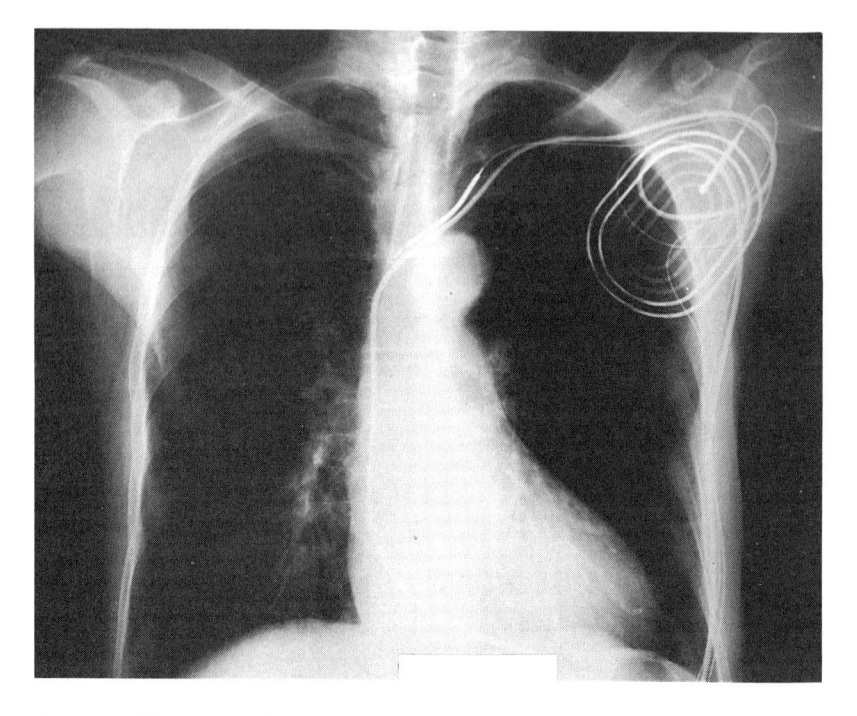

Figure 3. *Chest x-ray showing the subcutaneous patch electrode in the pectoral position.*

whom decremental energy testing was accomplished, the DFT was 15 J in two patients, 20 J in one patient, and 10 J in the fourth patient.

The two patients in whom the pectoral patch implantation was not possible received, respectively, a hybrid configuration with an extrapericardial patch (case 1) and a coronary sinus configuration (case 4), both with a 24 J DFT.

The five patients had no perioperative complications, were mobilized within 24 hours, and were discharged within eight days.

During a mean follow-up of 145±68 days, there was no mortality and no complications except a pectoral seroma in one case at the third week.

In two of the five cases, 73 successful interventions of the Pacer Cardioverter Defibrillator were reported: 66 ventricular tachycardia episodes were terminated by antitachycardia pacing (60) or low energy cardioversion (6) and seven episodes of VF were terminated.

Table 2
Implanted Electrode Configurations, Defibrillation Thresholds, and Interelectrode Resistances

						Mean Resistances**	
	Lead Configuration						
Patient				Pulse	DFT*	1	2
1	RV:	—	EP	SG	24	—	66
2	RV:	LS	PP	SIM	20	75	98
3	RV:	LS	PP	SQ	15	89	77
4	CS:	RV	AP	SQ	24	47	71
5	RV:	LS	PP	SQ	24	64	63
6	RV:	LS	PP	SQ	15	76	67
7	RV:	LS	PP	SQ	10	70	75

DFT: defibrillation threshold; *: stored energy; **: in Ohm, for pulse-1 and pulse-2 pathways; AP: apical patch; LS: left subclavian vein; PP: pectoral patch; EP: extrapericardial patch; RV: right ventricle; CS: coronary sinus; SIM: simultaneous; SQ: sequential; SG: single.

Conclusions

In conclusion, cardioverter-defibrillator implantation using a pectoral subcutaneous patch was possible in five of seven patients. It was not associated with specific local or general complications and it provided the advantage of reducing the number of incisions from three to two. Moreover, it demonstrated long-term efficacy by successfully terminating all spontaneous arrhythmia recurrences.

Acknowledgments: We are grateful to David Malamuth, Giovanni Moretti, and Marina Ferrari for their professional engineering assistance.

References

1. Bardy GH, Johnson G, Poole JE, et al: A simplified, single lead unipolar implantable transvenous cardioverter-defibrillator. Circulation 1992; 86(I):792. Abstract.
2. Callagen F, Accorti P, Scott S, et al: Dependence of current intensity on thoracic electrode location during nonthoracotomy defibrillation. Eur J C P E 1992; (II):A-105. Abstract.
3. Bardy GH, Hofer B, Johnson G, et al: Implantable transvenous cardioverter-defibrillators. Circulation 1993; 87:1152-1168.

11

Relationship between Acute Defibrillation Threshold and Therapy Outcome

M. Block, G. Breithardt

The defibrillation threshold (DFT), perhaps a magic word in the world of implantable cardioverter-defibrillators (ICDs), is of critical importance for effective device therapy. Uncertainties exist as to how precisely the DFT can and should be determined. What DFT can still be accepted to ensure proper defibrillation of the patient by the ICD? Could the rigorous testing needed to achieve exact determination of DFT during implantation be hazardous for the patient?

Definition

The DFT is usually defined as the minimal impulse energy that is needed to consistently defibrillate the heart. Instead of energy, the voltage or the current of the impulse has also been used as measure for the DFT. The relation between stored energy, delivered energy, (leading edge) voltage, and current of the defibrillation impulse is dependent on the capacitor storing the energy and the impedance of the lead system. Defibrillation energy is important if longevity of the ICD battery is of primary interest; defibrillation voltage is important for selection of the output capacitor; and defibrillation current is proba-

From *Transvenous Defibrillation and Radiofrequency Ablation* edited by A. John Camm and Fred W. Lindemans © 1995, Futura Publishing Co., Inc., Armonk, NY.

bly the most meaningful parameter from a physiological perspective. The DFT is usually assessed intraoperatively to ensure a sufficiently high defibrillation success rate with the amount of energy available in the implanted ICD.[1]

Defibrillation Dose-Response Curves

In pacing, there is only a small difference between the voltage (at a given pulse width) that consistently captures the heart and that which consistently does not. This difference is markedly larger in defibrillation. Therefore, the pacing dose-response curve is a step curve while the defibrillation dose-response curve has a sigmoidal shape (Fig. 1).[2] During pacing, only a few cells at the tip of the catheter have to be excited to initiate excitation of the whole myocardium. As the pacing stimulus usually is delivered when cells are not refractory, a reproducible starting point exists for every pacing stimulus. In contrast, defibrillation does not occur in relation to a trigger point of the cardiac cycle but occurs at random during fibrillation. The number of refractory and nonrefractory cells and their distribution within the nonhomogeneous defibrillation field differ with every defibrillation attempt. Therefore, the current needed to defibrillate a critical number of cells required for successful defibrillation differs from attempt to attempt.

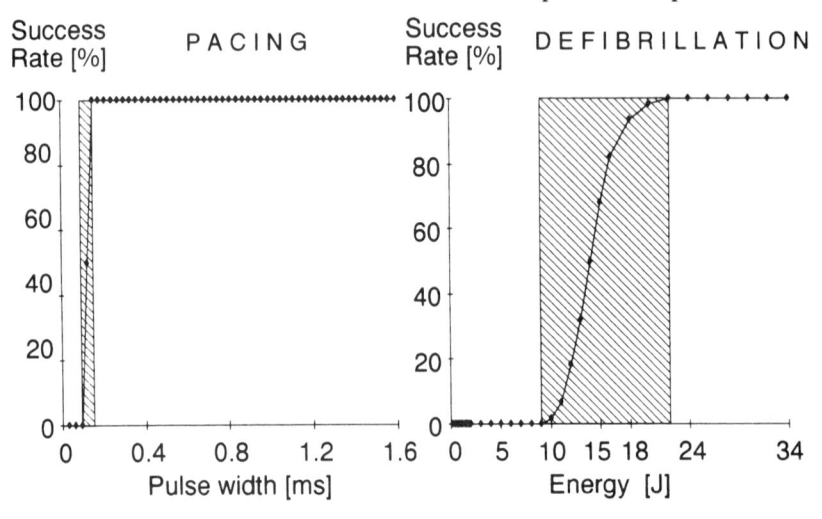

Figure 1. *Safety margin of defibrillation is lower compared to pacing. Hypothetical dose-response curves for pacing and defibrillation in comparison to the range of pacing pulse widths and defibrillation energies available in an ICD.*

Since defibrillation at a certain voltage may be successful at one time but may fail a next time, determination of DFT becomes a statistical problem. It is essential to know how many defibrillation trials and what energy levels are used to determine the DFT because the result of a DFT determination will depend on the test protocol used.

At least, the success rate of defibrillation at the maximal energy available in the ICD to be implanted should be sufficiently high to make the chance negligible that all consecutively available defibrillation therapies in the ICD would fail during a spontaneous episode of ventricular fibrillation (VF). Even in animal models, defibrillation dose-response curves can be only approximated since the number of VF episodes that can be reliably tested in one animal experiment is limited. In humans, true defibrillation dose-response curves cannot be obtained.[3] Curves obtained in dogs suggest that the difference between approximately 0% and 100% defibrillation efficacy shows a range in the order of 10 J.[2] Curves in different dogs differed in their DFT also in the order of 10 J and furthermore in the slope of their dose-response curve. An aggregate human defibrillation dose-response curve constructed from many patients by Church et al[4] showed a range from 300 V (approximately 5 J) to 900 V (approximately 50 J).

In internal defibrillation, at least some patients have shown failures at or even above the maximum energy available with ICDs. Therefore, it has been suggested that ICD implantation should not be performed without proper intraoperative testing of defibrillation energy requirements.

Determination of Defibrillation Thresholds in Humans

A step-down procedure in steps of approximately 5 J is frequently used, starting from, for example, 18 J or 24 J. Usually, the lowest successful energy in the step-down procedure is determined and sometimes incorrectly called the DFT. Some investigators have determined the DFT differently as they have continued to test until a minimal energy has been found at which three successful defibrillations are achieved without any failure. This approach prolongs DFT testing. Therefore, reconfirmation at the minimal successful energy level is used by many investigators only for 24 J or sometimes also 18 J. Figure 2 shows the range in which a hypothetical human defibrillation dose-response curve could be located if successful defibrillation at 24 J has

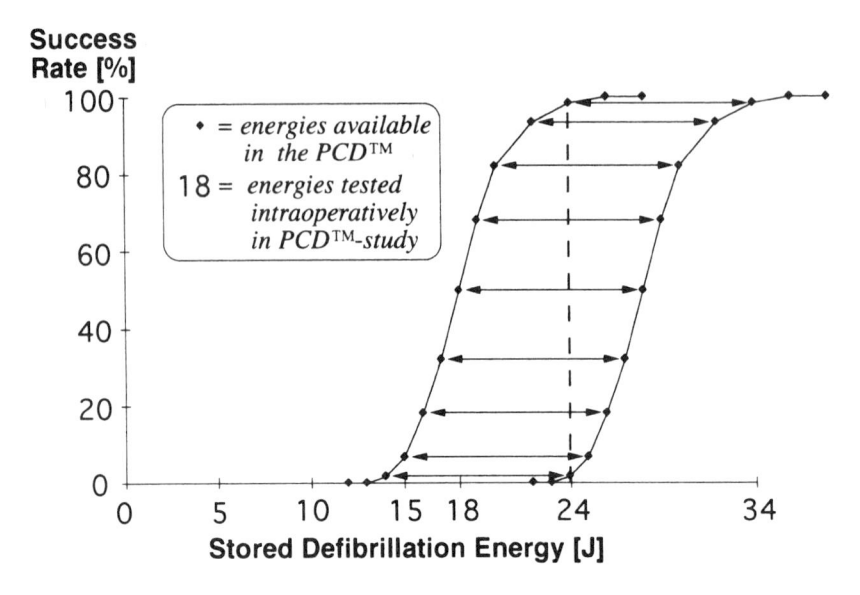

108 • TRANSVENOUS DEFIBRILLATION AND RF ABLATION

Figure 2. *Illustration of the high uncertainty of the patient's DFT with a single defibrillation success. If a single successful defibrillation with 24 J has been obtained, a hypothetical dose-response curve could be located within the range shown. The range of the hypothetical dose-response curve between 0% and 100% defibrillation efficacy is assumed to be 10 J.*

been achieved once. It illustrates the theoretical explanation for 10 J safety margin used by nearly all implanting centers. The margin of 10 J is also based on the relation between the intraoperative DFT and successful postoperative predischarge DFTs found by Marchlinski et al[5] in humans. They showed that only patients with an acute DFT of <10 J below the maximal energy available by the ICD showed failures of ICD discharges at the maximal energy available. Due to the limited number of VF episodes induced and the high energy or voltage steps used, a significant uncertainty about the real DFT remains if DFTs are measured in the clinical setting. More uncertainty exists about the true value of these DFT measurements as several investigators could show that these measurements are influenced by several variables and that DFT measurements were not completely stable if repeated after weeks to months.

Variables Influencing the Defibrillation Threshold

The variables that influence the DFTs are related to the patient, to the electrode system and the waveform used, and to the type of testing.

Patient-dependent variables might be relatively stable intraindividually like the volume of the heart or unstable like the medication of the patient. Wang and Dorian[6] showed that defibrillation energy requirements differed between anesthetic agents in dogs. No human data are available so far. Several studies exist showing that antiarrhythmic drugs frequently raise the DFT but might also decrease the DFT.[7] Sousa et al[8] showed that administration of epinephrine might significantly increase DFT.

In contrast to pacing and pacing thresholds, many defibrillation studies have shown that the shape of the waveform, for example, monophasic versus biphasic, has an impact on the DFT.[9] Also, the kind[10] and number of electrodes[8] used, their position, and their polarity[11] influence DFT results.

Winkle et al[12] have shown that the DFT rises with the duration of VF before defibrillation.

Short-Term and Long-Term Stability of Defibrillation Thresholds

In chronic animal experiments, the short-term (days to weeks) stability of DFT has been demonstrated.[13,14] In humans, most of the information on the stability of the DFT is derived from repeated DFT measurement during ICD replacements. Today, these results are only available for epicardial patches or the combination of an epicardial patch and a spring lead in the superior vena cava. Results from Wetherbee et al[15] indicate that no rise in DFT occurs with epicardial patches but might be seen if an intravenous spring lead is involved. Few results exist for transvenous (-subcutaneous) defibrillation systems obtained from DFT measurements in the electrophysiology laboratory before discharge or during follow-up of the patients. Preliminary results by Venditti et al[16] have shown a rise in DFT for transvenous or transvenous-subcutaneous defibrillation electrodes (Endotak™ by CPI). After two months, the DFT had risen by an average of 3 J, and after six months, it had risen by an average of 5 J.[16] For another transvenous or transvenous-subcutaneous defibrillation system (Transvene™ by Medtronic), preliminary results by Wathen et al[17] have shown a temporarily significant rise in DFT of 3 J at discharge from the hospital, but stable DFTs after six months. In contrast, Jung et al[18] reported preliminary results that indicated a 4 J improvement in DFT at discharge. Thus, short-term stability of DFTs of transvenous (-subcutaneous) defibrillation systems shows conflicting results in small studies, and long-term stability has still to be evaluated.

Complications of Defibrillation Threshold Testing

Perioperative morbidity and mortality have often been attributed to extensive perioperative DFT testing although convincing data to support this view have been lacking. Substantial improvements in perioperative morbidity and mortality with transvenous (-subcutaneous) defibrillation lead systems have led to abandonment of this hypothesis. During the introduction period of the new lead system, non-availability of biphasic defibrillation waveforms and conservative DFTs mandatory for final implantation (18 J or 20 J) led to extensive DFT testing by the primary investigators.[19] Despite this fact, a perioperative mortality of only about 1% was encountered in these studies. Studies have been performed to analyze the direct impact of DFT testing on cardiac and cerebral function. In patients who received epicardial patches via a thoracotomy approach, Hachenberg et al[20] found detrimental temporary effects on hemodynamics while others did not.[21] Winkle et al[12] could show that acute postshock hemodynamic depression was pronounced after long episodes of VF. In a study by Vester et al[22] during endocardial lead implantation, no prolonged or cumulative effects of DFT testing on hemodynamic functions were observed with intervals of at least 3 minutes between fibrillation episodes. In patients receiving epicardial defibrillation patches, no myocardial injury could be detected after DFT testing and spontaneous discharges up to cumulative energies of 330 J.[23] Singer et al[24] reported that no neurological damage was observed, though cerebral ischemic changes resulting from hypoperfusion during DFT testing persisted for hours if fibrillation episodes lasted longer than 30 seconds or more than six episodes were induced.

Relationship between Acute Defibrillation Threshold and Therapy Outcome

Intraoperative measurement of acute DFTs is done to ensure successful defibrillation during spontaneous episodes of ventricular tachyarrhythmias. The goal of ICD therapy is to prevent sudden cardiac death during follow-up. Sudden cardiac death with an implanted ICD is a rare event with annual rates of approximately 1% in long-term studies with epicardial defibrillating electrodes (Table 1)[25] and 0.2% in the first year of one multi-center study with transvenous (-subcutaneous) defibrillation electrodes (Table 2).[26] These excellent results were achieved in studies in which no patient received an ICD who showed constant intraoperative failure of defibrillation with the maximal energy available in the ICD to be implanted. Therefore, there is a lack of information on how an ICD would perform if it had been implanted despite excessively high DFTs. Of interest is the observation by Grubb et al[27] that, in six patients with epicardial patches, excessively high initial DFTs resolved at predischarge testing. In the study by Winkle et al,[25] three patients had no safety margin at implantation. In one of these patients, the ICD had to be explanted before hospital discharge

Table 1
Distribution of Acceptable and Unacceptable Acute DFTs and Resulting ICD Implantations in One Large Single Center ICD Study with Epicardial Leads. Sudden Cardiac Death Rate in the Study after One Year

DFT	Defined	Safety Margin	% of Patients Tested n = 273	Implanted n = 270
≤25 J	acceptable	≥5 J	98%	99%
>25 J	unacceptable	none	2%	1%
Sudden cardiac deaths at 1 year (188 patients): 1%				

DFT: defibrillation threshold. Source: Winkle RA, et al.[25]

Table 2
Distribution of Acceptable and Unacceptable Acute DFTs and Resulting ICD Implantations in One Large Multicenter ICD Study with Endocardial Leads. Sudden Cardiac Death Rate in the Study after One Year

DFT	Defined	Safety Margin	% of Patients* Tested n = 854	Implanted n = 757
≤18 J	acceptable	>10 J	64%	72%
= 24 J	unacceptable	= 10 J	33%	22%
>24 J	unacceptable	<10 J		2%
Sudden cardiac deaths at 1 year (113 patients): 0.2%				

DFT: defibrillation threshold; *: in some patients, DFT was not determined.
Source: Medtronic Model 7217B PCD™ Transvene™ Lead System report of October 27, 1992.

because it was found to accelerate ventricular tachycardia (VT) to VF that it could not terminate. Other patients reported by Winkle et al[25] had a safety margin of <10 J but sudden cardiac deaths during follow-up were attributed by the authors to other reasons than high acute DFTs. Pinski et al[28] reported that they found high DFTs (≥25 J) in 18% of their patients with epicardial lead systems. Eighteen patients received an ICD despite high DFTs. During a follow-up of 22±11 months, two patients died suddenly. In the world-wide Transvene™ experience, nearly all patients in whom an ICD was implanted had a safety margin of >10 J. Comparing patients with a safety margin of 10 J and >10 J, no differences could be shown for sudden cardiac death rates (Table 3). On one hand, a higher sudden cardiac death rate might be expected with a lower safety margin at implantation as DFT values are influenced by uncontrollable variables such as catecholamine levels and might rise with time. On the other hand, spontaneous VF during follow-up will be treated by at least four shocks in a row, but primary VF is a rare event. In contrast, VT requires less energy for termination. Failures of the first or even third shock will not cause sudden cardiac death but are undesirable as they could cause syncope and related injuries. As third generation devices allow differentiation among the success rates for first, second, third, and fourth defibrillation attempts, an analysis can be performed relating acute DFTs to the number and order of failing ICD discharges. Since such an analysis has not yet been done, we retrospectively looked for this possible relationship.

Between September 4, 1989 and January 27, 1993, 95 patients received a PCD™ at our institution. During implantation, the minimal successful defibrillation energy was determined by a step-down proce-

Table 3
Relation between Acute DFT and Therapy Outcome during Follow-up in One Large Multi-center ICD Study with Endocardial Leads

DFT	≤18 J	= 24 J
Number of patients	543	170
Mean follow-up	6 months	4 months
VF episode efficacy	99%	100%
Sudden cardiac deaths	n = 3	n = 1
One year sudden cardiac death survival	100%	99%

DFT: defibrillation threshold; VF: ventricular fibrillation.
Source: Medtronic Model 7217B PCD™ Transvene™ Lead System report of October 27, 1992.

dure (24 or 18 J, 15 J, 10 J, 5 J) in 71 patients. All patients were discharged with the maximal energy of 34 J programmed for all available therapies for fast ventricular tachyarrhythmias. During a mean follow-up of 16 (range: 0 to 40) months, 236 episodes of fast (average: 200 beats/minute) VT/VF within the VF-zone of the PCD™ were treated in 37 patients. Tachycardias were classified as ventricular based on algorithms using available electrocardiographic documentation and information from the RR interval memory of the PCD™. Figure 3 shows how often the first, second, third, and fourth shock was successful in terminating VT/VF in relation to the maximal failing energy during implantation. There was a clear tendency that more shocks of second, third, or fourth order were required with higher maximal failing energies during intraoperative testing. In patients who had intraoperative failures at 18 J or higher, 12 of 47 shocks (26%) delivered during spontaneous VT/VF failed. In patients who had maximal failing energies of <18 J, only 18 out of 218 shocks (8%) failed ($P \le .001$). The only patient who died suddenly during follow-up had no detection of a spontaneous tachycardia episode.

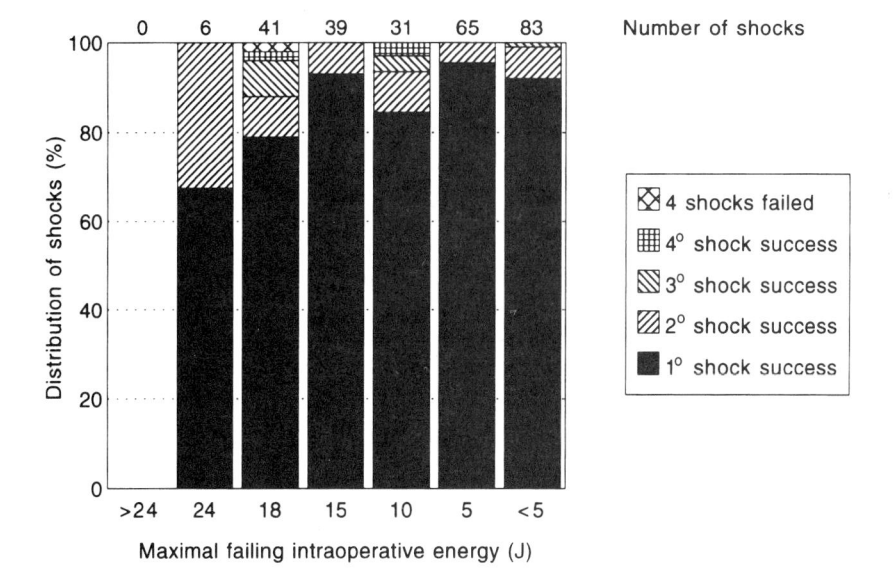

Figure 3. *Relation between acute DFT (represented by maximal failing defibrillation energy) and number of failing cardioversions/defibrillations (with 34 J) during spontaneous VT/VF in 37 patients with a PCD™.*

Is Defibrillation Threshold Testing Still Mandatory?

Long-term follow-up of ICD patients with epicardial patches as well as short-term follow-up of patients with transvenous (-subcutaneous) leads has shown that sudden cardiac death is a rare event after implantation of an ICD. These results have been established nearly exclusively for patients in whom intraoperative DFTs had been at least 10 J below the maximal energy of the implanted ICD. If initial DFTs resulted in smaller safety margins, leads were usually repositioned until this goal of ≥10 J safety margin was achieved.

Though no relationship has been found between the occurrence of sudden cardiac death and acute DFTs, such a relationship might appear if failures of defibrillation at or near the maximal energy of the ICD were analyzed. Our analysis has clearly demonstrated that patients near the 10 J safety margin needed significantly more shocks to terminate spontaneous fast VTs or VF than patients with a higher safety margin.

DFT testing seems to be a safe procedure; no correlation between the amount of intraoperative testing and perioperative morbidity and mortality has been reported. Intraoperative hemodynamic and electroencephalographic studies have established recommendations as to how DFT testing should be performed in order to minimize temporary suppression of hemodynamics and cerebral function. All electrophysiologists performing DFT testing are encouraged to change waveform, polarity, and number or position of leads until sufficient defibrillation is achieved.

Implantations without a thoracotomy have a substantially lower perioperative morbidity and mortality than implantations involving thoracotomy. Therefore, the decision to change to epicardial patches if successful defibrillation cannot be achieved with endocardial leads will increase the risk of the procedure. This has led to the development that during investigational implantations of endocardial leads, the necessary DFT was raised from the more conservative levels to the 10 J rule established for epicardial patches (Endotak™: 15 J → 20 J → 25 J; Transvene™: 18 J → 24 J). Since small studies have shown that the DFT of endocardial leads might rise during short-term follow-up, no higher intraoperative DFT should be accepted until the impact of these changes of testing procedure have been evaluated over long-term follow-up.

Determination of the "true DFT" is not mandatory for routine implants, but effective defibrillation about 10 J below the maximal energy of the device should be ensured. Determination of lower DFTs could enable the physician to program less energy for defibrillation or perhaps, in the future, to use a device with less maximal energy. A lower defibrillation energy can be delivered by the ICD in a shorter time and may prevent syncope in more patients. ICDs with a lower maximal energy could have a reduced size and might more easily be implanted subpectorally.

Conclusion

No relationship between acute DFTs and sudden cardiac death rates has been established. Retrospective analyses of large ICD data bases to establish such a relationship are not available. Prospective studies including patients with inadequate defibrillation at the maximal energy output of the implanted device or without any DFT testing cannot be justified as no data are available showing that DFT testing is dangerous, and long-term survival free of sudden cardiac death is excellent with current intraoperative testing procedures.

References

1. Block M, Borggrefe M, Hammel D: Intraoperative testing for defibrillator implantation. In LJ Kappenberger, FW Lindemans (eds.): Practical Aspects of Staged Therapy Defibrillators. Mount Kisco, NY, Futura Publishing Co, 1992, pp. 11-15.
2. Gliner BR, Mrakawa Y, Thakor N: The defibrillation success rate versus energy relationship: Part I—Curve fitting and the most efficient defibrillation energy. PACE 1990; 13:326-328.
3. Gliner BE, Mrakawa Y, Thakor N: The defibrillation success rate versus energy relationship: Part II—Estimation with the "bootstrap". Pace 1990; 13:425-431.
4. Church T, Martinsson M, Kallok M, et al: A model to evaluate alternative methods of defibrillation thresholds determination. PACE 1988; 11:2002-2007.
5. Marchlinski FE, Flores B, Miller J, et al: Relation of the intraoperative defibrillation threshold to successful postoperative defibrillation with an automatic implantable defibrillator. Am J Cardiol 1988; 62:393-398.
6. Wang M, Dorian P: Defibrillation energy requirements differ between anaesthetic agents. J Electrophysiol 1989; 3:86-94.
7. Block M, Lubienski A, Böcker D, et al: The use of antiarrhythmic drugs in patients with antitachycardia-cardioverter-defibrillator systems. In M Santini, M Pistolese, A Alliegro (eds.): Progress in Clinical Pacing 1992. Mount Kisco, NY, Futura Media Services Inc, 1993, pp. 95-112.

8. Sousa J, Kou W, Calkins H, et al: Effect of epinephrine on the efficacy of the internal cardioverter-defibrillator. Am J Cardiol 1992; 69:509-512.
9. Block M, Hammel D, Böcker D, et al: Biphasic shock waveform and a single bipolar transvenous lead should be the nonthoracotomy defibrillation of first choice. Circulation 1992; 86(I):442. Abstract.
10. Troup PJ, Chapman PD, Ollinger GN, et al: The implanted defibrillator: Relation of defibrillating lead configuration and clinical variables to defibrillation threshold. J Am Coll Cardiol 1985; 6:1315-1321.
11. O'Neill PG, Kwabena AB, Lawrie GM, et al: The automatic implantable cardioverter-defibrillator. Effect of patch polarity on defibrillation threshold. J Am Coll Cardiol 1991; 17:707-711.
12. Winkle RA, Mead RH, Ruder MA, et al: Effect of duration of ventricular fibrillation on defibrillation efficacy in humans. Circulation 1990; 81:1477-1481.
13. Fain ES, Billingham M, Winkle RA: Internal cardiac defibrillation: Histopathology and temporal stability of defibrillation energy requirements. J Am Coll Cardiol 1987; 9:631-638.
14. Kallok MJ, Olson WH, Marcaccini SJ, et al: Temporal stability of sequential pulse defibrillation threshold. PACE 1986; 9:1361-1366.
15. Wetherbee JN, Chapman PD, Troup PJ, et al: Long-term internal cardiac defibrillation threshold stability. PACE 1989; 12:443-450.
16. Venditti FJ, Vassolas G, Martin D: Chronic defibrillation thresholds in an implanted transvenous cardioverter defibrillator system. Circulation 1992; 86(I):441. Abstract.
17. Wathen M, Yee R, Klein G, et al: Chronic defibrillation threshold for automatic cardioverter defibrillator. PACE 1992; 15(II):1. Abstract.
18. Jung W, Manz M, Moosdorf R, et al: Relation of intraoperative to postoperative defibrillation threshold in patients with a nonthoracotomy lead system. J Am Coll Cardiol 1992; 19:242A. Abstract.
19. Block M, Hammel D, Isbruch F, et al: Results and realistic expectations with transvenous lead systems. PACE 1992; 15:665-670.
20. Hachenberg T, Hammel D, Möllhoff T, et al: Cardiopulmonary effects of internal cardioverter/defibrillator implantation. Acta Anaesthesiol Scand 1991; 35:626-630.
21. Antunes ML, Spotnitz HM, Livelli FD Jr, et al: Effect of electrophysiological testing on ejection fraction during cardioverter/defibrillator implantation. Ann Thorac Surg 1988; 45:315-318.
22. Vester EG, Winter J, Schipke J: Einfluss der seriellen Testung der Defibrillationsschwelle auf die linksventrikuläre Funktion während ICD-Implantation. Herzschr Elektrophys 1991; 2:164. Abstract.
23. Avitall B, Port S, Gal R, et al: Automatic implantable cardioverter/defibrillator discharges and acute myocardial injury. Circulation 1990; 81:1482-1487.
24. Singer I, Edmonds H, Slater D, et al: Cerebral hypoperfusion is an important factor to consider when programming implantable defibrillators. PACE 1992; 15(II):530. Abstract.
25. Winkle RA, Mead RH, Ruder MA, et al: Long-term outcome with the automatic implantable cardioverter defibrillator. J Am Coll Cardiol 1989; 13:1353-1361.
26. Model 7217B PCD™ Transvene™ Lead System Report of October 27, 1992.

27. Grubb BR, Marcini M, Temesy-Armos P, et al: Resolution of high initial epicardial patch defibrillation thresholds following chronic implantation. PACE 1992; 14:149-151.
28. Pinski SL, Vanerio G, Castle LW, et al: Patients with a high defibrillation threshold: Clinical characteristics, management and outcome. Am Heart J 1991; 122:89-95.

12

Chronic Clinical Results of Nonthoracotomy Implantable Cardioverter-Defibrillator Therapy

J. Brachmann, L.D. Sterns, T. Beyer,
W. Schoels, T. Hilbel, H. Mehmanesh,
R. Lange, J. Ruf-Richter, W. Saggau, K. Seidl,
S. Hagl, W. Kübler

The effectiveness of implantable cardioverter-defibrillator (ICD) therapy for the prevention of sudden death in patients with potentially lethal ventricular tachyarrhythmias has been evaluated in a number of studies. In the last several years, the development of nonthoracotomy lead systems has increased the ease of insertion of these devices and has potentially increased their indications for use in patients with ventricular arrhythmias. With earlier use of these devices often being considered over medical therapy, long-term device results should be very closely scrutinized, not only with regard to prevention of sudden cardiac death but also to consideration of the efficacy of arrhythmia discrimination and termination, device complications, and overall survival.

The results presented in this chapter are based on the experience with ICD therapy using transvenous/subcutaneous electrode systems

From *Transvenous Defibrillation and Radiofrequency Ablation* edited by A. John Camm and Fred W. Lindemans © 1995, Futura Publishing Co., Inc., Armonk, NY.

in the hospital of the Ruprechts-Karls University in Heidelberg and in the municipal hospital of Ludwigshafen.

Patient Population

Between February, 1990 and November, 1992, 75 patients were intraoperatively assessed for implantation of a Medtronic Model 7217 Pacer-Cardioverter-Defibrillator (PCD™) device using the Transvene™ lead system. These patients included 62 male and 13 female patients, with a mean age of 58±13 years, with a range from 19 to 77 years. Forty-five patients had coronary artery disease, 18 had dilated cardiomyopathy, 3 had long QT syndrome that was refractory to conventional medical therapy, and 9 had other implant indications.

Success Rate of Transvenous Implantation

The primary success rate of implanting the transvenous system was 92%: i.e., 69 of the 75 patients in whom a nonthoracotomy implantation was attempted could receive the system. The remaining six patients required an additional epicardial patch lead, in all cases due to inadequately high defibrillation thresholds (DFT >24 J). The successful implantations had a mean DFT of 18.1±4 J. The number of patients failing nonthoracotomy implantation will likely be reduced in the future with the availability of devices with biphasic defibrillation waveforms.

All patients except one received a system consisting of two transvenous leads and a subcutaneous patch. The right ventricular active fixation lead contained the pace-sense lead and its combined high energy coil was connected to the negative "common" terminal of the ICD. The second lead was a single high energy coil located in the superior vena cava (SVC) that was connected to the positive pulse-1 terminal of the device, and the third lead was a subcutaneous patch electrode connected to the positive pulse-2 terminal. In one young female patient with congenital heart disease, implant criteria were met with a single shock pathway between the right ventricular (cathode) and SVC (anode) electrodes.

Implantable Cardioverter–Defibrillator Programming

The mean tachycardia detection interval selected in these patients was 401 milliseconds, with a range of 330 to 530 milliseconds. The long detection intervals were required in a few patients with slow ventricular tachycardias (VTs) who typically present a challenge with regard to the inappropriate detection of fast ventricular rhythms during atrial fibrillation (AF). Present detection mechanisms do not always provide a safe solution for resolving this problem. The number of intervals to detect the tachycardia was programmed to 12 in all patients and the interval stability criterion was not used in any of them. The mean fibrillation detection interval was programmed to 319 milliseconds with a range from 270 to 370 milliseconds.

Ventricular tachycardia therapies were programmed "on" in 44 of the 69 patients (64%). The first VT therapy was antitachycardia pacing therapy in 36 patients and cardioversion in the remaining 8. Therapies for ventricular fibrillation (VF) were all programmed at 34 J, which is the maximum output of the device.

Spontaneous Episodes

All patients were followed for a minimum of one year except in the case of death before this time. Mean follow-up was 21.5 months, with the longest duration being of 43 months. In the first year, 52% of the devices detected and treated at least one episode of VF, and 66% of the devices detected and treated VF within two years. These numbers include only those episodes felt clinically to be true VF and do not include inappropriate detections of sinus tachycardia or supraventricular arrhythmias. Of the 44 patients with VT therapy programmed "on," 75% of these devices detected and treated an appropriate VT in the first year and 78% of these devices detected and treated VT by the end of the second year.

The differentiation between ventricular and supraventricular arrhythmias remains a difficult problem with these devices, as often both may occur in the same patient at nearly the same rate.

Therapeutic Efficacy

During the complete follow-up period, 34 of 44 patients with VT therapies programmed "on" were determined to have appropriately detected episodes of VT. These patients had a total of 1505 spontaneous VT episodes, of which 1346 (89.4%) were effectively treated with the first tachycardia therapy, and 1461 (97.1%) were cumulatively termi-

Therapy of Spontaneous VT Episodes

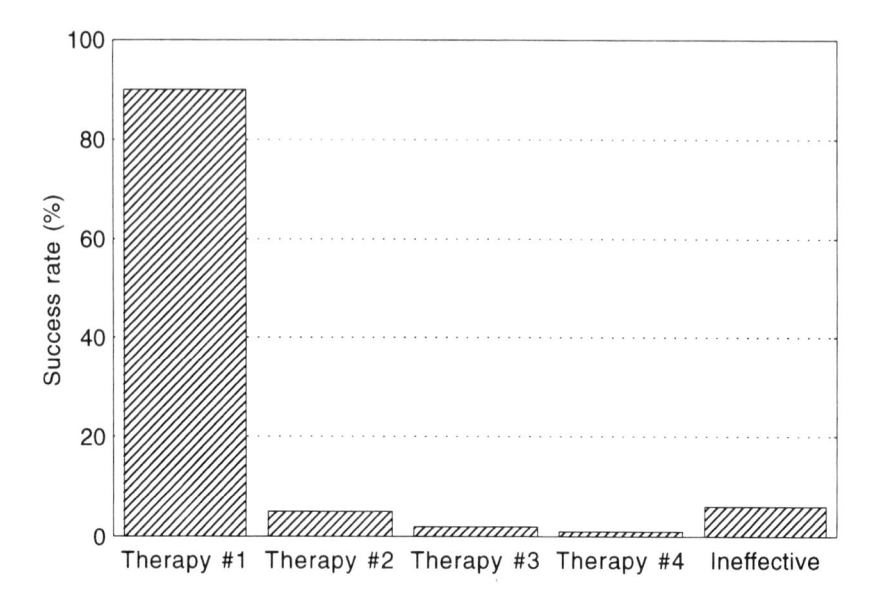

Figure 1. *Total number of spontaneous VT episodes and their termination by subsequent VT therapies.*

nated by the end of the fourth therapy (Fig. 1). In 31 of these patients, antitachycardia pacing was programmed as the first therapy. In these cases, the first therapy successfully terminated the tachycardia in 1294 of 1448 episodes, or in 89.3%.

Of the total patient group, 43 were determined to have appropriately detected episodes of VF. These patients had a total of 528 episodes, of which 457 were successfully terminated with the first defibrillation therapy for an efficacy of 86.6% for the first shock. All episodes were successfully terminated by the fourth therapy (Fig. 2). One patient suffered a sudden cardiac death 14 months after device insertion. Following his collapse, he was taken to a separate center and the device was never interrogated. If his death was considered a result of ineffectively treated VF, the efficacy of VF therapy would still be 99.8%.

Complications

Although the ICD device has proven to be very successful in terminating spontaneous VT and VF episodes, several problems with

Therapy of Spontaneous VF Episodes

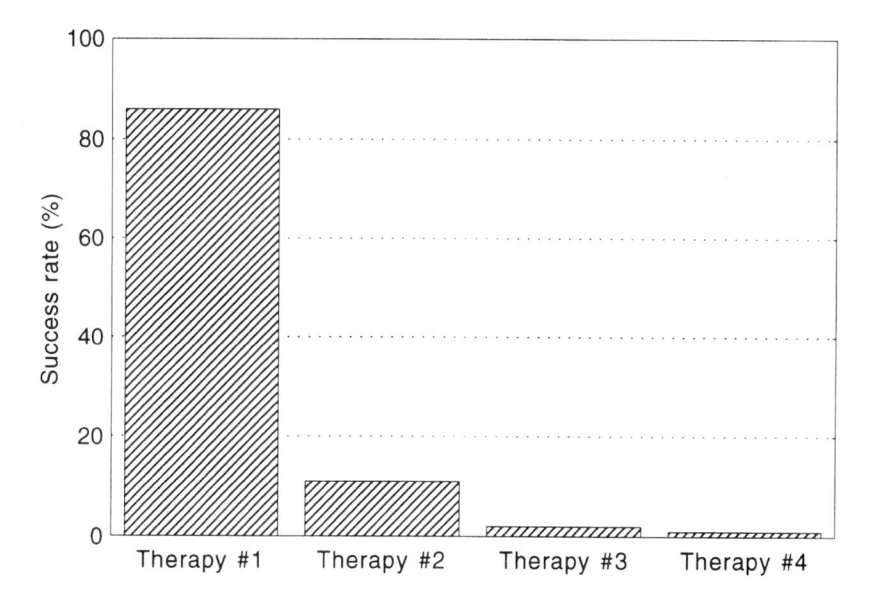

Figure 2. *Total number of spontaneous VF episodes and their termination by subsequent VF therapies.*

the device still exist and need resolution. These can be divided into those related to the implantation and those related to the device itself. Of implant-related problems, the most prevalent was hematoma formation at the site of the subcutaneous patch. This was usually minor and did not require operative drainage. In several of these cases, the hematoma occurred in patients requiring anticoagulation because of prosthetic valves or chronic AF and may have been related to too rapid reinitiation of heparin following the implantation. This will likely be minimized in the future with the decreasing need for subcutaneous patches with the new biphasic waveform devices. While no infections or implant-related mortality occurred with the initial device insertion in any of these patients, one patient died of sepsis following generator replacement.

One of the major device-related problems as pointed out above is the false detection of supraventricular arrhythmias leading to inappropriate therapy delivery. Although in our series there were no observed deleterious effects of these therapies besides the psychological stress of the shocks, they have been reported to induce real and potentially lethal ventricular arrhythmias in some cases, representing true device

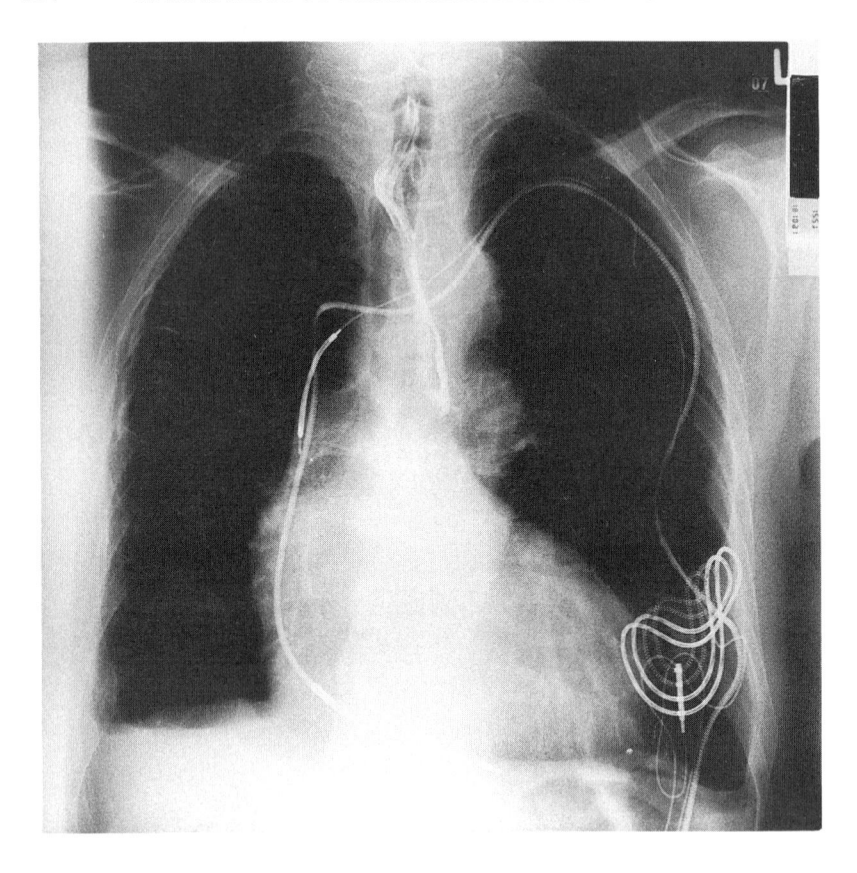

Figure 3A. *Posteroanterior chest x-ray showing patch crinkling that significantly raised the DFT and required operative correction.*

"proarrhythmia." When false detections were observed, medications were added to slow atrioventricular node conduction and/or device reprogramming was performed to decrease the chance of further inappropriate therapies.

The other significant device-related complication was lead fracture or dislocation and patch "crinkling." Figures 3A and 3B show posteroanterior and lateral chest x-rays of a patient in whom the subcutaneous patch developed a marked folding during chronic follow-up. This not only led to marked discomfort for the patient, but also caused a significant increase in DFT that required re-operation. In total, three patients required re-operation for patch crinkling (one required re-operation two times), three required re-operation for right ventricular lead dislocation (two within the first month), and three required re-operation for SVC

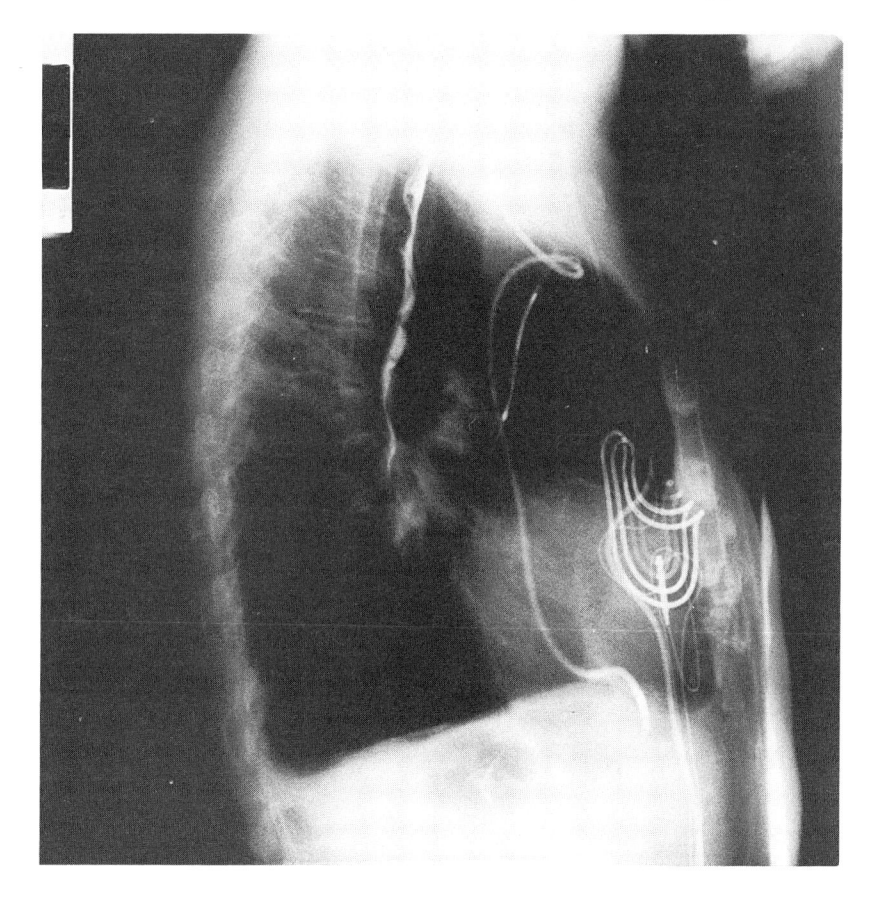

Figure 3B. *Lateral chest x-ray showing patch crinkling that significantly raised the DFT and required operative correction.*

lead displacement. The majority of the intravascular lead dislocations occurred within the first three months after implantation, whereas the patch crinkles all occurred later than 10 months postimplant.

Overall Survival

During follow-up, only 1 of the 69 patients with a transvenous/ subcutaneous lead system suffered a sudden cardiac death, occurring 14 months after device implantation. Total cardiac mortality in the group at one year was 7.3%, and at two years was 10.5%. Total mortality was 10.1% at one year, and 21.1% at two years. Figure 4 shows the

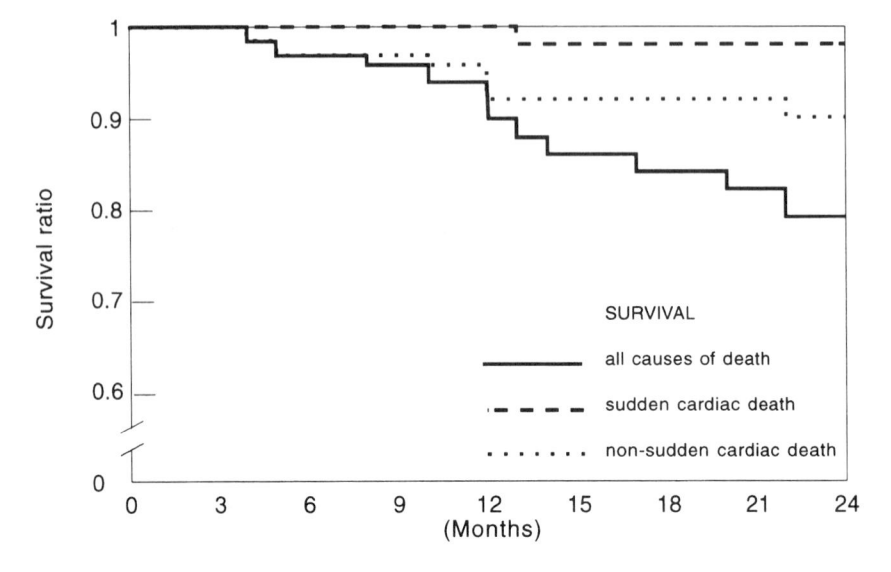

Figure 4. *Actuarial survival curves for 69 patients with a transvenous/subcutaneous lead system.*

actuarial survival curves for these patients with regard to sudden death, nonsudden cardiac death, and total mortality.

Conclusions

From these data, we can make the following observations, as detailed below.

1. The combination of antitachycardia pacing, low energy cardioversion, and high energy defibrillation therapy in one device provides a highly effective technique for the treatment of malignant ventricular tachyarrhythmias.
2. Nonthoracotomy implantation systems appear to have less surgical morbidity and mortality than the older epicardial systems while maintaining excellent protection against sudden arrhythmic death.
3. Dislocation of transvenous electrodes remains a major problem that hopefully will be improved by new electrode technologies. Subcutaneous patch problems are also presently a significant cause of postoperative morbidity and need for re-operation.
4. Differentiation of atrial and ventricular tachyarrhythmias continues to be the major functional problem with the device. New

technologies such as atrial sensing electrodes, hemodynamic sensors, or ventricular morphometric signal analysis will hopefully improve arrhythmia discrimination in the future.
5. Additional technical developments, such as the introduction of biphasic shocks for reduction of DFTs and the reduction of generator size, will soon allow the exclusive use of endocardial leads, mostly without subcutaneous patch electrode, and subpectoral implantation of the ICD device. This will simplify the surgical effort and reduce morbidity and discomfort for the patient.

The present generation of ICDs with nonthoracotomy lead systems continues to prove its reliability in the detection and treatment of malignant ventricular arrhythmias and prevention of sudden arrhythmic death. While future technical advances will improve the ease of insertion and accuracy of therapy of these devices, utilization studies now must focus on improving patient selection and possibly increasing prophylactic use in high-risk patients.

13

Treatment of Ventricular Tachycardia with Antitachycardia Pacing in Patients with an Implantable Cardioverter-Defibrillator

J. Siebels, R. Rüppel, M.A.E. Schneider, K.-H. Kuck

Since the first application of the implantable cardioverter-defibrillator (ICD) in humans by Michel Mirowski[1] in 1980, the first two generations of ICDs terminated ventricular tachyarrhythmias by either cardioversion or defibrillation. Sudden death mortality could be reduced to 1% to 2% per year by implantation of an ICD in a patient population at high risk for sudden arrhythmic death.[2,3]

Defibrillation of ventricular fibrillation (VF) is usually painless because of loss of consciousness or presyncope of the patient prior to shock delivery. In contrast, cardioversion of a hemodynamically stable ventricular tachycardia (VT) is painful for the majority of patients and involves a risk of acceleration of VT to VF.[4] Since antitachycardia pacing for treatment of VT proved to be highly effective in selected patient populations, antitachycardia pacemakers were developed and tested in patients with recurrent sustained VTs who were suitable for this treatment.[5-8] Because of the risk of acceleration from monomorphic VT

From *Transvenous Defibrillation and Radiofrequency Ablation* edited by A. John Camm and Fred W. Lindemans © 1995, Futura Publishing Co., Inc., Armonk, NY.

to polymorphic tachycardia or VF, backup defibrillation for antitachycardia pacing was required.

Since 1989, third generation ICDs with cardioversion, defibrillation, and antitachycardia pacing have become available. These devices offer many different modes and settings for antitachycardia pacing in addition to cardioversion and defibrillation. However, to test all different types of antitachycardia pacing modalities is time consuming and often uncomfortable for the patient. The efficacy of antitachycardia pacing in a large ICD patient population with a history of VT, syncope, and cardiac arrest is unknown.

The objectives of the study were to answer the following questions, as listed below.

1. Is a universal antitachycardia pacing mode in patients with an ICD effective and safe for the treatment of VTs?
2. Are there any differences with regard to the effectiveness of antitachycardia pacing in induced and spontaneous VTs?
3. Does antitachycardia pacing carry any risk by prolonging ischemia until definitive treatment is delivered?

Methods

This study was performed in patients with an implanted pacemaker-cardioverter-defibrillator (Medtronic, model 7216 or 7217 PCD™), which allows the testing of two different autoadaptive antitachycardia pacing modes for VT termination:

Ramp

- decreasing stimulation interval within attempt
- increasing number of stimulation pulses between attempts

Burst

- fixed stimulation interval within attempt
- fixed number of stimulation pulses
- decreasing stimulation interval between attempts

The PCD™ allows a maximum of four consecutive VT therapies with either Ramp, Burst, or Cardioversion (0.2 to 34 J). In case of failure in terminating the tachycardia with the programmed number of sequences of VT therapy #1, the device continues with VT therapy

#2, and so on. If the tachycardia is not terminated after delivery of all four VT therapies, the device is disabled for further therapy of the ongoing tachycardia. For VF therapy, the PCD™ allows four independent subsequent defibrillations with 0.2 to 34 J.

In this study, all patients were programmed to antitachycardia Ramp pacing, which allows the following therapeutic options:

tachycardia coupling interval: 97% to 50%

decrement per pulse: 10 to 50 milliseconds

number of pulses: 1 to 15

number of sequences: 1 to 15

minimum stimulation interval: 150 to 300 milliseconds

All patients with a history of spontaneous or inducible monomorphic tachycardia during preoperative electrophysiological (EP) study were tested prior to hospital discharge. A "universal" Ramp pacing for treatment of VT was programmed to the following parameters:

tachycardia coupling interval: 81%

number of initial pulses: 3

decrement per pulse: 10 milliseconds

minimum coupling interval: 200 milliseconds

number of sequences: 4 to 5

The VT detection interval was programmed between 440 and 320 milliseconds and the VF detection interval was programmed between 320 and 250 milliseconds. If tachycardia was reproducibly inducible with the telemetric programmed stimulation of the ICD, this Ramp was tested at least three times in each patient. If tachycardia was not inducible during predischarge testing, the same Ramp was programmed empirically for treatment of spontaneous tachycardia episodes. The "universal" Ramp was changed when, during ICD testing, an induced VT was not changed at all and a consecutive cardioversion was necessary for termination of tachycardia. In case of acceleration (≥40 milliseconds) of VT to a more rapid monomorphic or a polymorphic tachycardia or to VF during predischarge testing, the Ramp parameters were not changed. In all patients with the VF detection programmed <300 milliseconds, reproducible detection and termination of VF was tested to ensure that VF was properly detected and treated without interference with the VT detection.

Testing was performed in the EP laboratory under mild to moderate intravenous sedation with midazolam (5 to 10 mg) or diazepam (5 to 10 mg).

Follow-up was performed one month after surgery, followed by visits every three months or after spontaneous ICD discharges with complete interrogation of the ICD. The PCD™ features two different arrhythmia episode and therapy data registers for VT and VF. These include four counters each with the number of successful treatments (VT therapy #1-4, VF therapy #1-4). These counters allow the analysis of successful Ramp therapies as well as accelerations caused by the therapies when the success counter for the VT therapy has not been incremented while the VF therapy counter has been incremented.

During follow-up, acceleration of a tachycardia can be detected only if acceleration above the VF cutoff rate occurs. For analysis in this study, a tachycardia was interpreted as accelerated when the interval record of the device showed a VT therapy before VF detection, when acceleration was documented, or when acceleration was suspected because long episodes of palpitations followed by defibrillation were reported by patients with usually long tachycardia cycle lengths.

The PCD™ allows an exact analysis of tachycardia cycle length only for the last VT or VF episode. Therefore, the mean cycle lengths cannot be analyzed for all spontaneous tachycardias. All spontaneous tachycardia episodes in which atrial arrhythmias with rapid atrioventricular conduction occurred were excluded from the analysis.

Results

Until June, 1992, 59 patients (56±13 years, 12 female, 47 male) received the PCD™. The underlying heart disease was coronary artery disease in 39 patients, dilated cardiomyopathy in 14, and other diseases in 6 patients. The mean left ventricular ejection fraction was 34%±13%. Forty of the 59 patients had a history of documented sustained monomorphic VT or inducible tachycardia during preoperative EP testing. In 26 of the 40 patients, a total of 94 monomorphic VTs treated with Ramp was induced during predischarge ICD testing. Table 1 lists the efficacy as well as the risk of tachycardia acceleration with respect to patients as well as tachycardia counts.

In three patients, the tachycardia coupling interval of the Ramp sequence had to be shortened to 75% due to ineffective antitachycardia pacing of all episodes with subsequent cardioversion of the unchanged tachycardia. The mean cycle lengths of the terminated, unchanged, or

Table 1
Efficacy of RAMP Pacing for Ventricular Tachycardia during Predischarge Testing

	Termination n (%)	No Change n (%)	Acceleration n (%)
Ventricular tachycardias	73 (78)	5 (5)	16 (17)
Patients*	15 (58)	—	11 (42)
VT cycle length (ms)	326±44	330±44	308±56

*: at least one tachycardia accelerated to VF therapy; VT: ventricular tachycardia

accelerated tachycardias as well as the patient characteristics in the three groups did not differ.

During a mean follow-up of 14±11 months in 20 of the 26 patients with inducible VT and in 10 of the 14 patients without inducible tachycardia, a total of 1248 spontaneous VT episodes occurred. Table 2 lists the efficacy of Ramp pacing for VT during follow-up with respect to patients and tachycardia counts.

Only 2 of the 11 patients with acceleration of tachycardia due to Ramp pacing at the ICD test had acceleration of tachycardia during follow-up. Two of 14 spontaneous tachycardias (14%) in one patient were accelerated to rapid tachycardia or VF and were terminated by defibrillation. In the second patient, one of the six (17%) tachycardias was accelerated due to antitachycardia pacing and required defibrillation. One additional patient without inducible VT at the ICD predischarge test had acceleration of 2 of the 13 (15%) tachycardias to rapid polymorphic tachycardia during follow-up (Table 2). None of the patients with acceleration of induced tachycardia during EP testing had

Table 2
Efficacy of RAMP Pacing for Ventricular Tachycardia during Follow-up

	Termination n (%)	No Change n (%)	Acceleration n (%)
All VT [all RAMP*] (1248 VT)	1184 (94.9)	59 (4.7)	5 (0.4)
VT [universal RAMP 3/81]	1037 (96.6)	35 (3.3)	1 (0.1)
Patients with inducible VT	19 (90)	—	2 (10)
Patients without inducible VT	8 (92)	—	1 (8)

*: including tachycardia coupling interval of 75% and 81% and different number of pulses; VT: ventricular tachycardia

acceleration of spontaneous tachycardias during follow-up. With regard to the total number of spontaneous tachycardias, the acceleration rate of the "universal" Ramp and all types of Ramp pacing was low (Table 2). The per patient number of tachycardia accelerations due to antitachycardia pacing was higher (about 15%).

Analysis of the tachycardia cycle length from the ICD data was possible in 16% of tachycardias during follow-up. Twenty-eight percent of the spontaneous tachycardias had rates between 200 and 250 beats/minute and Ramp pacing had similar success rates in these rapid tachycardias compared to tachycardias with rates below 200 beats/minute. No patient died due to Ramp pacing and tachycardia acceleration during follow-up.

One patient with 114 previously successfully treated tachycardias by Ramp pacing died suddenly after 13 months. The device counter reported one additional VF episode that was not terminated with four VF therapies (34 J) despite an intraoperative defibrillation threshold of 3 J. Failure for defibrillation probably occurred due to an insulation defect of one patch electrode with leakage of current to the generator.

Discussion

Several studies have demonstrated high success rates of antitachycardia pacing during EP testing in selected patient populations with hemodynamically stable VTs.[5-8] Various studies have revealed that autodecremental pacing with decreasing pacing intervals within a single attempt (Ramp) has the highest success rate during EP testing. Due to the lack of backup defibrillation, long-term studies with implanted antitachycardia pacemakers have been limited to patients with extremely low risk for acceleration of VT by pacing. The combination of separate antitachycardia pacemakers and ICD treatment has been limited due to interaction between ICD detection and antitachycardia pacing.

Since 1989, ICDs with antitachycardia pacing, cardioversion, and defibrillation have been available. Porterfield et al[9] reported a patient with a PCD™ supposedly having terminated 90 of 96 VT episodes with antitachycardia pacing within one week. A rather aggressive Ramp sequence with 84% coupling interval and 10 initial pulses had been programmed. However, a technical disadvantage of the device counters makes this high success rate in the reported patient unlikely: the PCD™ counts every tachycardia that is accelerated to the VF-zone and terminated by defibrillation (VF therapy) as a success for VF therapy and VT therapy. In addition to the 96 VT episodes, 23 VF episodes were reported within one week. In the worst case analysis, 23 of the 90 "successful" Ramp treatments could have been accelerations (26%).

Den Dulk et al[10] first investigated a universal mode of antitachycardia pacing for VT. The universal Ramp in our study was programmed to a quite aggressive coupling interval but featured a small number of stimuli to maximize efficacy while minimizing the risk of acceleration.

To exclude subselection of patients with a low risk of tachycardia acceleration, this study was performed in all consecutive patients with PCD™ implantation and previous or inducible VT regardless of tachycardia cycle length and acceleration during ICD testing.

During predischarge testing, the success rate of the tested universal Ramp protocol in this unselected patient population was lower than other pacing modes in highly selected patient populations.[7,8] In these studies, the authors postulated up to 100 successfully treated tachycardia events during preimplant EP testing before selection for implantation of a antitachycardia pacemaker. The high acceleration risk of at least one VT in 42% of patients in this study (Table 1) was much lower during follow-up (Table 2). The success rate of all types of Ramp pacing and especially of the universal Ramp during follow-up was extremely high, whereas the acceleration risk was extremely low. Analyzing the three patients with acceleration of tachycardias during follow-up demonstrated that 15% of tachycardias were accelerated in these patients due to Ramp pacing. At the time of acceleration, two of the three patients had progressed in their heart failure status from New York Heart Association (NYHA) II to NYHA III. In this study, only a small percentage of tachycardias was not changed by Ramp pacing and needed cardioversion for termination during follow-up (Table 2). As previously suspected, the PCD™ did not allow the exact number of accelerations of tachycardias to the VF-zone and VF therapy to be counted. In this study, there are several patients who have different documented tachycardias with different cycle lengths that exceeded the VF detection cutoff and were treated with VF therapy. If the worst case analysis is calculated in these patients, there were 37 undocumented VF episodes reported by the counters in addition to successful tachycardia treatments. If all VF episodes were VT accelerations, the risk of acceleration by Ramp pacing would have been about 3.5% of all spontaneous tachycardias, which is low for this population.

The discrepancy between the high acceleration rate of Ramp pacing during predischarge testing (17%) and during follow-up (0.4% to 3%) might be explained by differences in induced and spontaneous tachycardias. Modulating factors such as high autonomic tone and ischemia due to repeated tachycardia induction during predischarge testing might have influenced the efficacy of antitachycardia pacing significantly.

Conclusion

The findings of this study have several clinical implications. First, Ramp pacing with a coupling interval of 81% and three pulses with an incremental number of pulses between each attempt seems to be a universal antitachycardia pacing mode for most patients with an implanted defibrillator and spontaneous VTs. Second, acute testing of antitachycardia pacing in this patient population has a low predictive value. Antitachycardia pacing (Ramp) might be programmed regardless of accelerations during acute testing. Third, excessive testing of antitachycardia pacing before implantation of antitachycardia pacemakers is not necessary.

References

1. Mirowski M, Reid PR, Mower MM, et al: Termination of malignant ventricular arrhythmias with an implanted automatic defibrillator in human beings. N Engl J Med 1980; 303:322-324.
2. Winkle RA, Mead RH, Ruder MA, et al: Long-term outcome with the automatic implantable cardioverter-defibrillator. J Am Coll Cardiol 1989; 13:1353-1361.
3. Edel TB, Maloney JD, Moore S, et al: Six-year clinical experience with the automatic implantable cardioverter defibrillator. PACE 1991; 14:1850-1854.
4. Siebels J, Geiger M, Schneider MAE, et al: Implantable cardioverter/defibrillator—the potential hazard of programmability. Circulation 1990; 82(III):548. Abstract.
5. Fisher JD, Mehra R, Furman S: Termination of ventricular tachycardia with bursts of rapid ventricular pacing. Am J Cardiol 1978; 41:94-102.
6. Josephson ME, Horowitz LN: Electrophysiological approach to therapy of recurrent sustained ventricular tachycardia. Am J Cardiol 1979; 43:631-642.
7. Griffin JC, Sweeney M: The management of paroxysmal tachycardias using the Cybertach-60. PACE 1987; 7:1291-1295.
8. Rothman MT, Keefe JM: Clinical results with Omni-Orthocor, an implantable antitachycardia pacing system. PACE 1984; 7:1306-1312.
9. Porterfield JG, Porterfield LM, Bray L: Ninety-six episodes of spontaneous ventricular tachycardia in 1 week: Success of Ramp pacing by a Pacer-Cardioverter-Defibrillator. PACE 1991; 14:1440-1443.
10. Den Dulk K, Brugada P, Kersschot I, et al: Is there a universal anti-tachycardia pacemaker mode? PACE 1986; 9:302. Abstract.

14

The Use of Antiarrhythmic Drugs in Implantable Cardioverter-Defibrillator Patients

W. Jung, M. Manz, B. Lüderitz

The implantable cardioverter-defibrillator (ICD) has proven to be a safe and effective electrotherapeutic tool in the management of patients with life-threatening ventricular tachyarrhythmias.[1] Ideally, the ICD might eliminate the necessity for antiarrhythmic therapy after device implantation. However, up to 70% of patients who receive an ICD will also be maintained on concomitant antiarrhythmic drug treatment for a variety of reasons. Regarding the role of antiarrhythmic drugs in ICD patients, the following questions remain unresolved.

1. Is the widespread use of antiarrhythmic drug treatment in ICD recipients necessary?
2. Does antiarrhythmic drug therapy decrease the number of appropriate ICD therapies?
3. Is antiarrhythmic drug treatment in ICD patients associated with a greater chance of survival?

Thus, it is important to have an understanding of the potential interaction between the ICD and antiarrhythmic therapy. Several of

From *Transvenous Defibrillation and Radiofrequency Ablation* edited by A. John Camm and Fred W. Lindemans © 1995, Futura Publishing Co., Inc., Armonk, NY.

Table 1
Possible Interactions between Antiarrhythmic Drugs and Implantable Cardioverter-Defibrillator Systems

Proarrhythmic events, thereby increasing the number of shock deliveries.

Slowing of intraventricular conduction, which might lead to double counting or to satisfaction of PDF criteria for VT.

Alterations in DFT.

Increase or decrease in VT cycle length that can influence the effectiveness of antitachycardia pacing.

Change from sustained to nonsustained VT, resulting in inappropriate shocks during nonsustained VT.

Alteration in postshock excitability.

Increase in pacing thresholds.

DFT: defibrillation threshold; PDF: probability density function; VT: ventricular tachycardia

the possible interactions of antiarrhythmic medications with the ICD are listed in Table 1.

Effects of Antiarrhythmic Drugs on the Defibrillation Threshold

Most of our knowledge of the effects of antiarrhythmic drugs on defibrillation threshold (DFT) is based on animal data.[2-6] Table 2 provides an overview of the impact of various antiarrhythmic agents on DFT. The Class IC agents encainide, flecainide, and propafenone have uniformly demonstrated adverse effects on DFTs. It has been shown that encainide increases the energy required for 50% successful defibrillation in open chest anesthetized dogs by 129±43%.[7] Flecainide and propafenone have been reported to elevate defibrillation energy requirements in a dog model.[8,9] In contrast to the Class IC drugs, Class IA agents, which have less of an effect on sodium conductance, may not significantly alter the energy requirement for defibrillation if used in therapeutic doses. Several investigators have reported that quinidine or procainamide did not change DFTs.[10,11]

Table 2
Effects of Antiarrhythmic Drugs on Defibrillation Thresholds

Increase	No Change	Decrease
Encainide	MODE	Sotalol
ODE	Quinidine	
Propafenone	Procainamide	
Flecainide		
Lidocaine		
Mexiletine		
Amiodarone		Amiodarone
(chronic)		(acute)

MODE: 3-methoxy-O-desmethylencainide; ODE: O-desmethylencainide

The Class IB agent lidocaine has been demonstrated to cause a dose-dependent increase in defibrillation energy requirements in an animal model.[12] A recently published report suggested that these adverse effects may be related to an anesthetic lidocaine interaction.[13] Another Class IB drug, mexiletine, has been associated with an increase in DFT in a single patient.[14]

A decrease in DFT has been recently reported for the newer Class III agent sotalol.[15] Application of intravenous sotalol significantly reduced the energy requirements for successful defibrillation in anesthetized dogs. The effect of amiodarone, another Class III agent, on DFT has been controversial and may be dependent on duration of therapy and route of drug administration.[16-21] Animal data are inconsistent and frequently differ from clinical experience. In dogs, it was shown that the energy required for successful defibrillation is decreased by an acute administration of intravenous amiodarone, while chronic oral administration had no significant effect.[16] While intravenous amiodarone has been shown to have beneficial effects in patients who had either an out-of-hospital cardiac arrest or prolonged resuscitation, oral administration of amiodarone seems to elevate energy requirements for successful defibrillation.[17-24]

In order to evaluate the long-term stability of internal defibrillation energy requirements, a prospective study of DFTs at the time of implantation and generator replacement was conducted in 22 patients using a patch/patch epicardial configuration.[22] The concomitant antiarrhythmic drug treatment consisted of either mexiletine (720 mg/day) or amiodarone (400 mg/per day) and was administered to patients in a randomized and parallel manner. During a mean follow-up period of 24±6 months, the DFT increased significantly from 14.3±2.8 J to 17.9±5.3

J ($P<0.05$) for the entire patient group. The increase in the chronic DFT was due to a marked increase in defibrillation energy needs in the subgroup of patients receiving amiodarone. No significant change in the DFT was documented in the subgroup of patients receiving mexiletine. The mean DFT increased from 14.1±3.0 J to 20.9±5.4 J ($P<0.001$) in those receiving amiodarone. In all patients with increased DFTs, the reevaluation showed a reduction in the DFT after discontinuation of the antiarrhythmic drug therapy. The only variable associated with the increase in the chronic DFT was amiodarone treatment.[22-24] It therefore appears that amiodarone given acutely will lower the DFT while, in contrast, it may elevate it when given chronically.

Effects of Antiarrhythmic Drugs on Arrhythmia Recognition by the Implantable Cardioverter-Defibrillator

Antiarrhythmic drugs may have other clinically significant effects that can potentially have an impact on the arrhythmia recognition by the ICD. Antiarrhythmic drugs may increase latency or cause PR interval prolongation or QRS widening. This may result in double counting if diastolic signals are oversensed. Figure 1 shows an example of intermittent double counting at the highest sensitivity during monomorphic ventricular tachycardia (VT) in a patient who received chronic amiodarone therapy. After discontinuation of amiodarone, the phenomenon of double sensing disappeared. Alterations in QRS morphology or interventricular conduction delay may result in a morphology that is indistinguishable from VT during supraventricular tachycardia or atrial fibrillation. In such a case, inappropriate shock delivery may result if the rate of the tachycardia exceeds the cutoff rate of the device. Solutions to this problem include incorporation of an atrial sensor and/or a hemodynamic sensor.[2]

Antiarrhythmic Therapy for Slowing of Ventricular Tachycardia

The Class I antiarrhythmic agents as well as the Class III agents produce slowing of conduction. Procainamide and amiodarone will each produce a mean increase in VT cycle length of approximately 25% when a morphology identical to that observed in the baseline state is

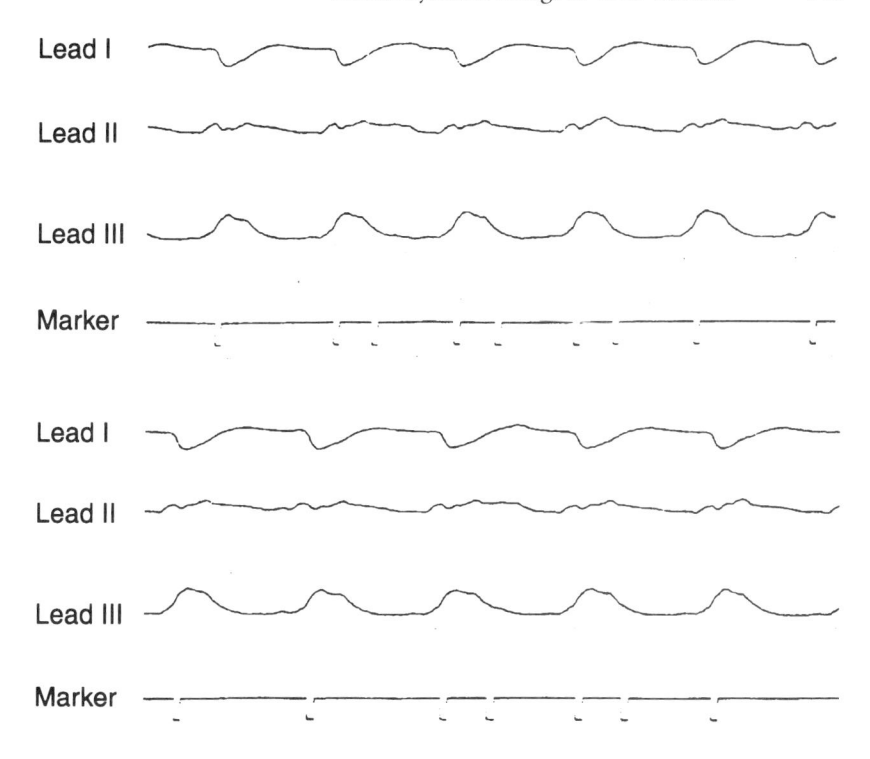

Figure 1. *In a patient receiving chronic amiodarone therapy, intermittent double counting was noted at the highest sensitivity level during monomorphic VT. Lead I, II, III: surface electrocardiogram leads; Marker: event marker.*

reinitiated.[25,26] Mexiletine generally has less of an effect on tachycardia cycle length. Earlier defibrillator generations were not programmable in terms of their algorithm for tachycardia detection. This concern for nondetection has been virtually eliminated by the present programmable features of more sophisticated devices. However, electrophysiological (EP) testing may still be mandatory to define tachycardia cycle length and thereby ensure adequate tachycardia detection if the institution of antiarrhythmic agents is deemed necessary after implantation. The slowing of VT that is observed with antiarrhythmic agents may have several beneficial effects. There appears to be a significant relationship between tachycardia cycle length and the ability to terminate VT with antitachycardia pacing.[27-31] Tachycardias that are relatively slow are more easily terminated by pacing or programmed simulation and may be less prone to tachycardia acceleration.[3]

Alteration in Postshock Excitability and Increase in Pacing Thresholds

Shock delivery of an ICD may cause a change in the amplitude of endocardial electrograms and impair the detection of ventricular fibrillation (VF).[32,33] In patients with a nonthoracotomy lead system, failure of an ICD to redetect VF following an unsuccessful shock attempt has been recently described.[33] Beside postshock sensing problems, antiarrhythmic drugs may alter postshock tissue excitability leading to prolonged postdefibrillation pauses requiring pacing support. On the other hand, antiarrhythmic drugs may simultaneously elevate pacing thresholds resulting in the failure to capture postdefibrillation.[34-39] There are conflicting reports on the incidence of postdefibrillation bradycardia.[34,35] In addition, the effects of antiarrhythmic drugs on postshock pacing threshold have been controversially discussed.[36,39] Guarnieri et al[38] reported a temporary loss of ventricular capture following a 30 J ICD shock. The duration of capture loss was related to current strength and was significantly increased by the presence of Class IC antiarrhythmic drugs.[38] In contrast to these findings, a recently published report showed that ventricular pacing threshold was not significantly different from baseline values following an internal defibrillation shock of 20 J. In addition, the time to capture was short, and there was no significant difference in "no drug" versus amiodarone.[39]

Effects of Antiarrhythmic Drugs on the Incidence of Implantable Cardioverter-Defibrillator Shocks and on the Time Preceding the First Appropriate Implantable Cardioverter-Defibrillator Therapy

In a retrospective study, the effect of antiarrhythmic drug treatment on the incidence of ICD therapy was evaluated in 74 ICD recipients.[40] Thirty-three patients were treated with an antiarrhythmic drug that was either untested or was previously shown (during EP testing) to be ineffective in suppressing the induction of ventricular tachyarrhythmias. Forty-one patients were not treated with any antiarrhythmic drugs. The results of this study indicated that the length of time preceding an initial appropriate shock (5±5 months in both groups) and the frequency of ICD shocks were similar in both groups.[40] In addition, the study of Myerburg et al[41] showed no difference in the time preceding

Use of Antiarrhythmic Drugs in Implantable Cardioverter-Defibrillator Patients

The type of antiarrhythmic drugs used in our latest 101 ICD patients at the most recent follow-up is shown in Figure 2. Altogether, 90% of our patients were maintained on some kind of antiarrhythmic drugs including digitalis, β-blockers, and calcium antagonists. Only 10% of our patients were taken off all antiarrhythmic drugs. Half of our patients were treated with either Class I agents, Class III agents, or a combination of both. Amiodarone was prescribed to 10% of our patients. The indication for the use of antiarrhythmic agents is illustrated in Figure 3. Half of our patients received antiarrhythmic drugs to reduce the frequency of recurrent episodes of ventricular tachyarrhythmias. Approximately 20% of the patients were taking antiarrhythmic drugs to decrease the rate of spontaneous VTs in order to improve hemodynamic tolerance and to facilitate termination by antitachycardia

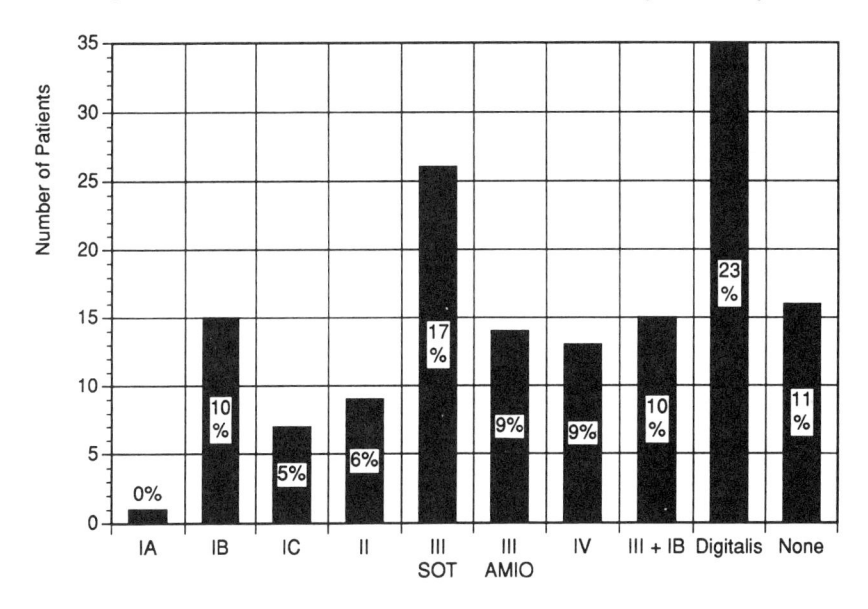

Figure 2. *Type and distribution of antiarrhythmic agent used in our latest 101 ICD recipients. I, II, III, IV: classification according to Vaughan Williams; Amio: amiodarone; Sot: sotalol.*

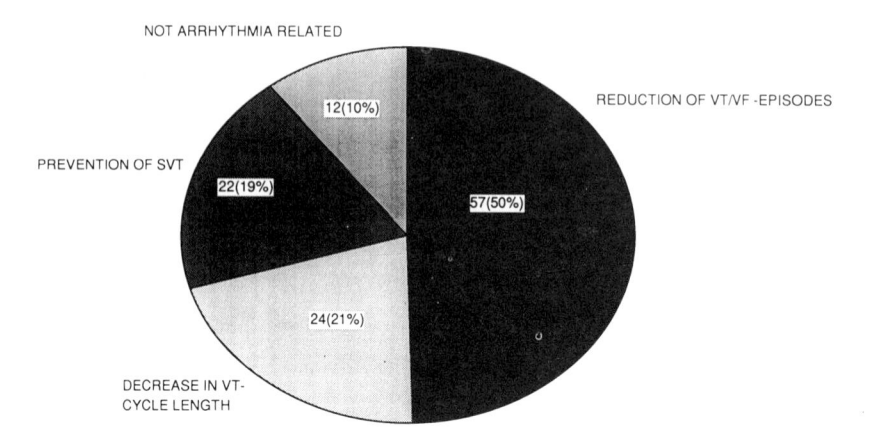

Figure 3. *Indications for the use of antiarrhythmic agents in our latest 101 patients with ICDs. SVT: supraventricular tachycardia; VF: ventricular fibrillation; VT: ventricular tachycardia.*

pacing. About 20% of the patients were treated with antiarrhythmic drugs in an attempt to control atrial tachyarrhythmias that might result in frequent inappropriate ICD discharges. In 10% of our patients, the use of antiarrhythmic drugs was not arrhythmia related.

Conclusions

Nowadays, antiarrhythmic drugs are used in the majority of patients with ICD systems. Based on the available data, there was no significant difference in the incidence of appropriate ICD therapy as well as in the length of time preceding a first appropriate ICD discharge between patients receiving antiarrhythmic drugs and those who did not. The findings do not provide strong evidence in favor of using antiarrhythmic drugs after an ICD implant in an attempt to reduce the frequency of ICD therapies and/or to prolong the time preceding a first ICD discharge. Further prospective and controlled studies will still be needed to establish the role of antiarrhythmic agents in ICD recipients.

References

1. Saksena S: Recent advances in implantable cardioverter-defibrillator therapy. In B Lüderitz, S Saksena (eds.): Interventional Electrophysiology. Mount Kisco, NY, Futura Publishing Co, 1991, pp. 395-414.

2. Singer I, Guarnieri T, Kupersmith J: Implanted automatic defibrillators: Effects of drugs and pacemakers. PACE 1988; 11:2250-2262.
3. Gottlieb CD, Horowitz LN: Potential interactions between antiarrhythmic medication and the automatic implantable cardioverter defibrillator. PACE 1991; 14:898-904.
4. Babbs CF: Alteration of defibrillation threshold by antiarrhythmic drugs. A theoretical framework. Crit Care Med 1981; 9:362-363.
5. Jung W, Manz M, Lüderitz B: Effects of antiarrhythmic drugs on defibrillation threshold in patients with the implantable cardioverter defibrillator. PACE 1992; 15:645-648.
6. Manz M, Jung W, Lüderitz B: ICD and antiarrhythmic drugs. In E Adornato, A Galassi (eds.): The '92 scenario in cardiac pacing. Rome, Italy, Edizioni Luigi Pozzi, 1992, pp. 141-143.
7. Fain ES, Dorian P, Davy JM, et al: Effects of encainide and its metabolites on energy requirements for defibrillation. Circulation 1986; 73:1333-1341.
8. Reiffel JA, Coromilas JM, Zimmermann JM, et al: Drug device interactions: Clinical considerations. PACE 1985; 8:369-373.
9. Peters W, Gang ES, Solingen A, et al: Acute effects of intravenous propafenone on the internal ventricular defibrillation energy requirements in the anaesthetized dog. J Am Coll Cardiol 1991; 17:129A. Abstract.
10. Dawson AK, Steinberg MI, Shapland JE, et al: Effects of class I and class II drugs on current and energy required for internal defibrillation. Circulation 1985; 72:III-383. Abstract.
11. Marchlinski FE, Flores B: Effect of procainamide on the defibrillation threshold in man. Circulation 1988; 78:II-154. Abstract.
12. Dorian P, Fain ES, Davy JM, et al: Lidocaine causes a reversible, concentration-dependent increase in defibrillation energy requirements. J Am Coll Cardiol 1986; 8:327-332.
13. Natale A, Jones DL, Kim YH, et al: Effects of lidocaine on defibrillation threshold in the pig: Evidence of anaesthesia related increase. PACE 1991; 14:1239-1244.
14. Marinchak RA, Friehling TD, Kline RA, et al: Effect of antiarrhythmic drugs on defibrillation threshold: Case report of an adverse effect of mexiletine and review of the literature. PACE 1988; 11:7-12.
15. Wang M, Dorian P: DL and D sotalol decrease defibrillation energy requirements. PACE 1989; 12:1522-1529.
16. Fain ES, Lee JT, Winkle RA: Effects of acute intravenous and chronic oral amiodarone on defibrillation energy requirements. Am Heart J 1987; 114:8-17.
17. Williams ML, Woelfel A, Cascio WE, et al: Intravenous amiodarone during prolonged resuscitation from cardiac arrest. Ann Intern Med 1989; 110:839-842.
18. Troup PJ, Chapman PD, Olinger GN, et al: The implanted defibrillator: Relation of defibrillating lead configuration and clinical variables to defibrillation threshold. J Am Coll Cardiol 1985; 6:1315-1321.
19. Fogoros RN: Amiodarone-induced refractoriness to cardioversion. Ann Intern Med 1984; 100:699-700.
20. Guarnieri T, Levine JH, Veltri EP, et al: Success of chronic defibrillation and the role of antiarrhythmic drugs with the automatic implantable cardioverter/defibrillator. Am J Cardiol 1987; 60:1061-1064.

21. Huang SKS, Tan de Guzman WL, Chenarides JG, et al: Effects of long-term amiodarone therapy on the defibrillation threshold and the rate of shocks of the implantable cardioverter-defibrillator. Am Heart J 1991; 122:720-727.
22. Jung W, Manz M, Pizzulli L, et al: Effects of chronic amiodarone therapy on defibrillation threshold. Am J Cardiol 1992; 70:1023-1027.
23. Jung W, Manz M, Pfeiffer D, et al: Effects of antiarrhythmic drugs on epicardial defibrillation energy requirements and the rate of defibrillator discharges. PACE 1993; 16:198-201.
24. Jung W, Manz M, Lüderitz B: Increase in chronic defibrillation threshold in patients with implantable cardioverter/defibrillator and additional drug therapy. New Trends Arrhyt 1992; 7:823-826.
25. Marchlinski FE, Buxton AE, Kindwall EK, et al: Comparison of individual and combined effects of procainamide and amiodarone in patients with sustained ventricular tachyarrhythmias. Circulation 1989; 78:583-587.
26. Vaitkus PT, Buxton AE, Josephson ME, et al: Cycle-length response of ventricular tachycardia associated with coronary artery disease to procainamide and amiodarone. Am J Cardiol 1990; 66:710-714.
27. Roy D, Waxman HL, Buxton AE, et al: Termination of ventricular tachycardia: Role of tachycardia cycle length. Am J Cardiol 1982; 50:1346-1350.
28. Naccarelli GV, Zipes DP, Rahilly GT, et al: Influence of tachycardia cycle length and antiarrhythmic drugs on pacing termination and acceleration of ventricular tachycardia. Am Heart J 1984; 107:638-643.
29. Keren G, Miura DS, Somberg JC, et al: Pacing termination of ventricular tachycardia: Influence of antiarrhythmic slowed ectopic rate. Am Heart J 1983; 105:1-6.
30. Lüderitz B: The impact of antitachycardia pacing with defibrillation. PACE 1991; 14:312-316.
31. Jung W, Manz M, Lüderitz B: Antiarrhythmic drug prescription for ICD patients. In LJ Kappenberger, FW Lindemans (eds.): Practical Aspects of Staged Therapy Defibrillators. Mount Kisco, NY, Futura Publishing Co, 1992, pp. 49-52.
32. Yee R, Jones DL, Klein GJ: Pacing threshold changes after transvenous catheter countershock. Am J Cardiol 1984; 53:503-507.
33. Jung W, Manz M, Moosdorf R, et al: Failure of an implantable cardioverter/defibrillator to redetect ventricular fibrillation in patients with a nonthoracotomy lead system. Circulation 1992; 86:1217-1222.
34. Platia EF, Griffith LSC, Reid PR, et al: Post-defibrillation bradycardia following implantable defibrillator discharge. J Am Coll Cardiol 1986; 7:144A. Abstract.
35. Niazi I, Kadri N, Mahmud R, et al: Absence of significant post defibrillation bradyarrhythmias in patients with automatic implantable defibrillators. Am Heart J 1988; 115:830-836.
36. Levick CE, Mizgala HF, Kerr CR: Failure to pace following high dose antiarrhythmic therapy—reversal with isoproterenol. PACE 1984; 7:252-256.
37. Hellestrand KJ, Burnett PJ, Milne JR, et al: Effect of the antiarrhythmic agent flecainide acetate on acute and chronic pacing thresholds. PACE 1983; 6:892-899.

38. Guarnieri T, Datorre SD, Bondke H, et al: Increased pacing threshold after an automatic defibrillator shock in dogs: Effects of class I and class II antiarrhythmic drugs. PACE 1988; 11:1324-1330.
39. Khastger T, Lattuca J, Aarons D, et al: Ventricular pacing threshold and time to capture postdefibrillation in patients undergoing implantable cardioverter-defibrillator implantation. PACE 1991; 14:768-772.
40. Kou WH, Kirsh MM, Bolling SF, et al: Effect of antiarrhythmic drug therapy on the incidence of shocks in patients who receive an implantable cardioverter defibrillator after a single episode of sustained ventricular tachycardia/fibrillation. PACE 1991; 14:1586-1592.
41. Myerburg RJ, Luceri RM, Thurer R, et al: Time to first shock and clinical outcome in patients receiving an automatic implantable cardioverter-defibrillator. J Am Coll Cardiol 1989; 14:508-514.

15

Transtelephonic Implantable Cardioverter-Defibrillator Monitoring

M.H. Anderson

The use of conventional telephone lines for the transmission of data from medical devices has a long history. Telephonic transmission of the electrocardiogram (ECG) was pioneered in the 1960s,[1] but a genuine practical use for such techniques was demonstrated by its early application to pacemaker follow-up. The mercury zinc cells used in early pacemakers displayed a very rapid voltage decline at the end of life and their longevity was unpredictable. To avoid very frequent clinic visits or the need for elective replacement of devices after an impractically short period, a system was developed to enable the transtelephonic transmission of pulses corresponding to magnet-triggered pacing output. By providing accurate measurement of changes in heart rate, it was possible to monitor pacemaker performance, thereby enabling elective replacement of the pacemaker just prior to battery exhaustion.[2]

Transtelephonic pacemaker follow-up has been widely used in the United States,[3] although less so in Europe. It is perhaps surprising that transtelephonic monitoring techniques did not develop in association with the development of early implantable defibrillators. The technical complexity of the device and its relatively rapid evolution may explain this occurrence.

From *Transvenous Defibrillation and Radiofrequency Ablation* edited by A. John Camm and Fred W. Lindemans © 1995, Futura Publishing Co., Inc., Armonk, NY.

150 • TRANSVENOUS DEFIBRILLATION AND RF ABLATION

Is Transtelephonic Interrogation Needed?

There has been a tendency to regard the implantable cardioverter-defibrillator (ICD) as merely a complicated pacemaker. However, this overlooks a fundamental difference between the devices. Pacemakers are designed to function as a "background" device. Satisfactory function of a pacemaker is not usually associated with symptoms. With the ICD, however, symptoms often continue despite the presence of the device, and the delivery of shock therapies by the device is readily noticed by the patient. The pattern of occurrence of symptoms and delivery of therapies may vary markedly with time and may give rise to uncertainty in the patient and physician over the correct functioning of the device. This uncertainty may require unscheduled clinic visits to enable interrogation of the device and to reassure the patient. The need for such unscheduled visits is likely to rise with the development of features such as automatic capacitor reform that reduces the need for frequent routine clinic visits. In countries where there are relatively few implanting centers or where the population is sparse, patients may have to undertake long journeys to the defibrillator clinic. At

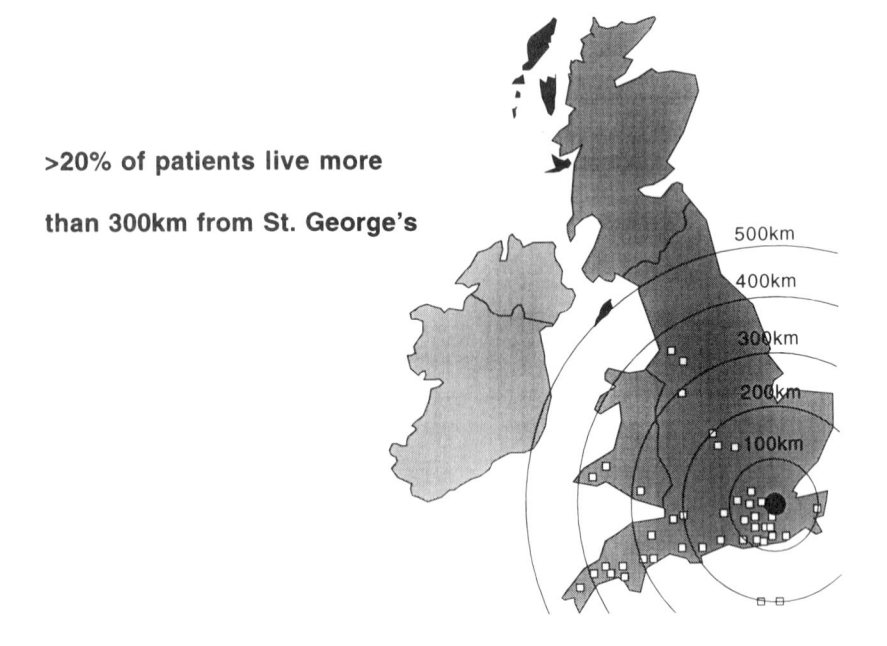

>20% of patients live more than 300km from St. George's

Figure 1. *Distribution of the 51 patients who have received the ICD at St. George's Hospital. Circles around London drawn with radius increasing in 100 km steps.*

Table 1
Potential Uses of Transtelephonic Implantable Cardioverter-Defibrillator Monitoring

Patient reassurance after therapy delivery
Reduction of clinic visits for routine checks
Datalog retrieval where storage is limited
Central follow-up of investigational devices

St. George's Hospital in London, our ICD patients live, on average, 120 km from the clinic, with some living over 500 km away (Fig. 1). These journeys are time consuming, expensive, and result in absence from work for patients who are keen to maintain their premorbid level of activity. If some visits to the clinic could be replaced by transtelephonic checks, disruption to patients' work could be minimized. It is also technically feasible to program the defibrillator by telephone and it might be useful to be able to make minor changes in pacing, detection, and therapy programming. However, it is doubtful whether the performance of pacing and sensing checks in the unsupervised home environment is safe or desirable. In devices like the Medtronic Model 72127 Pacer-Cardioverter-Defibrillator (PCD™) in which data storage is limited, transtelephonic interrogation enables data to be retrieved that would otherwise have been overwritten by the time of the patient's next clinic visit. Finally, future evaluation of new models of the ICD would involve much less administrative work and form completion if the manufacturer could interrogate the ICD directly in the patient's home or in the follow-up clinic. Potential uses of transtelephonic ICD monitoring are summarized in Table 1.

Current Transtelephonic Implantable Cardioverter-Defibrillator Monitoring Systems

Initial attempts to monitor the ICD by telephone involved the additional use of a continuously recording electrocardiographic monitor.[4] After therapy delivery, the patient could send the recorded ECG to the clinic for interpretation. The obvious drawback of this approach was the need for the patient to wear the electrocardiographic monitor at all times. This approach was only practical in the first few months after ICD implantation when the incidence of therapy delivery is higher.

152 • TRANSVENOUS DEFIBRILLATION AND RF ABLATION

The ability of some ICD generators to produce an R wave synchronized beep when in magnet mode has also been used to monitor sensing by telephone.

Only a small number of true transtelephonic interrogation devices has so far been developed for the ICD. The vast majority are single function devices designed either to indicate battery or device status. These have usually been developed in response to a specific need in investigational devices that have been shown to suffer from an unacceptably high incidence of premature battery depletion or spontaneous shutdown. They enable device integrity to be checked at a frequency that would be unacceptable to the patient if a hospital visit was involved.

The CPI Ventak PRx™ defibrillator has a limited transtelephonic interrogation capability that requires only the availability of a conventional transtelephonic electrocardiographic monitor. When transtelephonic mode is programmed to an active state, the application of a magnet over the device triggers a sequence of eight pacing pulses that are R wave synchronized. A second pacing pulse may follow the first at an interval of 100 milliseconds. The presence of a single or double pacing pulse is used as a simple binary code to convey device status information (Fig. 2).

Magnet triggered pacing pulses

These five pulses may be single or double
(100ms gap between double pulses)

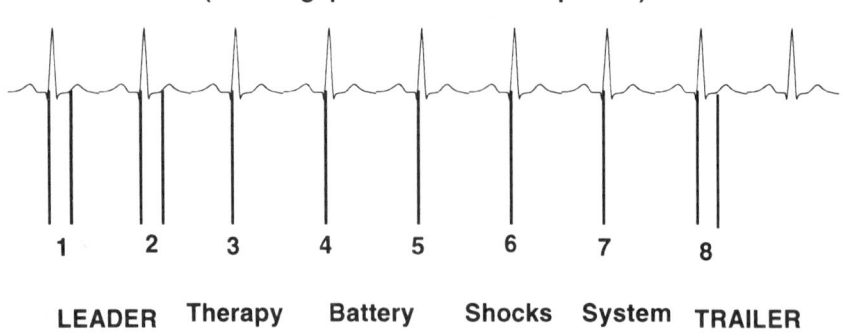

| 1 | 2 | 3 | 4 | 5 | 6 | 7 | 8 |

LEADER Therapy Battery Shocks   System   TRAILER
        On/Off   Status   Delivered Status

Figure 2. *The CPI Ventak PRx™ 1700 transtelephonic interrogation uses a sequence of eight magnet-triggered R wave synchronized pacing pulses. Pulses 3 to 7 may be single or double, and this binary code is used to transmit limited data on system status and performance.*

The Medtronic PCD™ Teletrace™ system (see Fig. 3) is currently the only one capable of full transtelephonic interrogation of an ICD. The system is a modification, produced for feasibility analysis, of the standard model 9421 Teletrace™ transmitter and model 9420 Teletrace™ receiver. These devices, designed for transtelephonic pacemaker follow-up, have been equipped with additional circuitry allowing interrogation of the PCD™ 7216A and 7217B defibrillators. The 9421 PCD™ Teletrace™ transmitter is powered by two 9 V batteries and is fully portable. Once telephone contact is established with the pacing clinic, the patient connects two elasticated metal bracelets to the transmitter and switches the transmitter on. The interrogation head is placed over the defibrillator and a light on the transmitter confirms correct placement. The patient places the telephone handset on the Teletrace™ transmitter and transmission commences automatically. Initially, a continuous tone transmits a short ECG rhythm strip, and this is followed by a series of fractionated tones lasting 50 seconds that convey the telemetry data. Finally, a continuous tone transmits an additional 20 seconds of ECG rhythm strip.

At the implanting center, the telephone receiver is placed on the Medtronic 9420 PCD™ Teletrace™ receiver as soon as the tones commence. The receiver is connected to a dot-matrix printer that produces a four page print-out identical in format to the output produced by the standard Medtronic programmer (Fig. 4). This print-out contains data on currently programmed backup pacing, ventricular tachycardia (VT) detection criteria, programmed VT therapies, ventricular fibrillation (VF) detection criteria, programmed VF therapies, battery status,

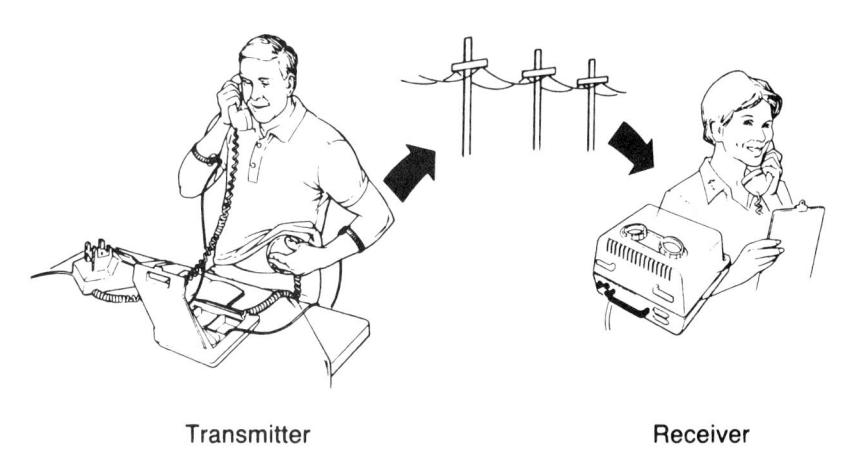

Figure 3. *Medtronic PCD™ Teletrace™ system.*

154 • TRANSVENOUS DEFIBRILLATION AND RF ABLATION

```
MEDTRONIC 9420PCD TELETRACE RECEIVER          MEDTRONIC 9420PCD TELETRACE RECEIVER
SOFTWARE REVISION: 9420PCD-002                SOFTWARE REVISION: 9420PCD-002
PCD MODEL 7216                                PCD MODEL 7216
TRANSMITTER ID: 00000355                      TRANSMITTER ID: 00000355

TIME AND DATE: 30-10-89  12                   TELEMETRY
                                              ---------
INTERROGATED VALUES:
                                              PERM TELEMETRY ENABLE            OFF
PACING AND SENSING                            TELEMETRY TYPE                   MRKR
------ --- -------
                                              DATA
   PACING MODE                    VVI         ----
   PACING RATE               50 PPM
   PACING PULSE WIDTH         1.01 MS         PCD STATUS:
   PACING AMPLITUDE            5.4 V             MEMORY RETENTION              OK
   SENSITIVITY                 0.6 MV            CHARGE CIRCUIT                OK
   REFRACTORY AFTER PACE      320 MS             LAST CHARGE TIME         3.04 SEC
                                                 CIRCUITRY BATTERY        3.04 V
VT DETECTION AND THERAPIES                       CHARGING BATTERY         6.49 V
-- ---------- --- ----------
                                              VT ONSET COUNTER                   0
VT DETECT:
   VT DETECTION ENABLE         ON             VT EPISODE AND THERAPY DATA:
   VT DETECTION INTERVAL      400 MS             EPISODE COUNT                   9
   # INTERVALS TO DETECT       12                VT THERAPY #1 SUCCESS COUNT     7
   INTERVAL STABILITY          60 MS             VT THERAPY #2 SUCCESS COUNT     2
   ONSET CRITERIA ENABLE      OFF                VT THERAPY #3 SUCCESS COUNT     0
   ONSET VALUE (R-R%)          81 %              VT THERAPY #4 SUCCESS COUNT     0
   ONSET COUNTER ENABLE       OFF                # OF VT'S PCD INEFFECTIVE       0
                                                 PCD EFFICACIOUS ON LAST VT    YES
VT THERAPY #1:                                   LAST THERAPY USED              #1
   THERAPY TYPE              RAMP%              #SEQ IN LAST PACE THERAPY        2
   VT THERAPY ENABLE          ON                R-R AVG FOR LAST PACE THRPY  320 MS
   INITIAL # OF S PULSES       4
   FIRST R-S INTERVAL          91 %           VF EPISODE AND THERAPY DATA:
   PER PULSE DECREMENT         10 MS             EPISODE COUNT                   6
   # OF SEQUENCES              2                 VF THERAPY #1 SUCCESS COUNT     4
   MINIMUM INTERVAL           200 MS             VF THERAPY #2 SUCCESS COUNT     2
                                                 VF THERAPY #3 SUCCESS COUNT     0
VT THERAPY #2:                                   VF THERAPY #4 SUCCESS COUNT     0
   THERAPY TYPE         CARDIOVERSION            # OF VF'S PCD INEFFECTIVE       0
   VT THERAPY ENABLE          ON                 PCD EFFICACIOUS ON LAST VF    YES
   CV PULSE WIDTH            6.3 MS              LAST THERAPY USED              #2
   CV ENERGY (JOULES)       20.1 JOUL
   CV CURRENT PATHWAY        SNGL


MEDTRONIC 9420PCD TELETRACE RECEIVER          MEDTRONIC 9420PCD TELETRACE RECEIVER
SOFTWARE REVISION: 9420PCD-002                SOFTWARE REVISION: 9420PCD-002
PCD MODEL 7216                                PCD MODEL 7216
TRANSMITTER ID: 00000355                      TRANSMITTER ID: 00000355

VT THERAPY #3:                                LAST EPISODE DETECTION SEQUENCE:
   THERAPY TYPE         CARDIOVERSION            -19. R-R INTERVAL-  750 MS
   VT THERAPY ENABLE          ON                 -18. R-R INTERVAL-  500 MS
   CV PULSE WIDTH            6.3 MS              -17. R-R INTERVAL-  600 MS
   CV ENERGY (JOULES)       34.1 JOUL            -16. R-R INTERVAL- 1110 MS
   CV CURRENT PATHWAY        SNGL                -15. R-R INTERVAL-  770 MS
                                                 -14. R-R INTERVAL-  670 MS
VT THERAPY #4:                                   -13. R-R INTERVAL-  360 MS
   THERAPY TYPE         CARDIOVERSION            -12. R-R INTERVAL-  570 MS
   VT THERAPY ENABLE          ON                 -11. R-R INTERVAL-  330 MS
   CV PULSE WIDTH            6.3 MS              -10. R-R INTERVAL-  320 MS
   CV ENERGY (JOULES)       34.1 JOUL             -9. R-R INTERVAL-  290 MS
   CV CURRENT PATHWAY        SNGL                 -8. R-R INTERVAL-  310 MS
                                                  -7. R-R INTERVAL-  300 MS
VF DETECTION AND THERAPIES                        -6. R-R INTERVAL-  300 MS
-- ---------- --- ----------                      -5. R-R INTERVAL-  310 MS
                                                  -4. R-R INTERVAL-  310 MS
VF DETECT:                                        -3. R-R INTERVAL-  310 MS
   VF DETECTION ENABLE        ON                  -2. R-R INTERVAL-  310 MS
   VF DETECTION INTERVAL     280 MS               -1. R-R INTERVAL-  320 MS
   # INTERVALS TO DETECT      18                  -0. R-R INTERVAL-  320 MS
                                                  -0. VT DETECTED
VF DEFIBRILLATION THERAPY #1:
   VF THERAPY ENABLE          ON             EVENTS AFTER LAST THERAPY:
   DEFIB PULSE WIDTH         6.3 MS              +0. VT THERAPY #1 DELIVERED
   DEFIB ENERGY (JOULES)    20.1 JOUL            +1. R-R INTERVAL-  920 MS
   DEFIB CURRENT PATHWAY     SNGL                +2. R-R INTERVAL-  300 MS
                                                 +3. R-R INTERVAL-  840 MS
VF DEFIBRILLATION THERAPY #2:                    +4. R-R INTERVAL-  720 MS
   VF THERAPY ENABLE          ON                 +5. R-R INTERVAL-  720 MS
   DEFIB PULSE WIDTH         6.3 MS              +6. R-R INTERVAL-  710 MS
   DEFIB ENERGY (JOULES)    34.1 JOUL            +7. R-R INTERVAL-  700 MS
   DEFIB CURRENT PATHWAY     SNGL                +8. R-R INTERVAL-  700 MS
                                                 +9. R-R INTERVAL-  710 MS
VF DEFIBRILLATION THERAPY #3:                   +10. R-R INTERVAL-  720 MS
   VF THERAPY ENABLE          ON                +10. THERAPY WAS SUCCESSFULL
   DEFIB PULSE WIDTH         6.3 MS           NO TELEMETRY DATA AVAILABLE
   DEFIB ENERGY (JOULES)    34.1 JOUL
   DEFIB CURRENT PATHWAY     SNGL

VF DEFIBRILLATION THERAPY #4:
   VF THERAPY ENABLE          ON
   DEFIB PULSE WIDTH         6.3 MS
   DEFIB ENERGY (JOULES)    34.1 JOUL
   DEFIB CURRENT PATHWAY     SNGL
```

Figure 4. *Medtronic PCD™ Teletrace™ print-out example.*

last charge time, episode counter and therapy log for VT and VF, and the RR intervals of the 20 beats preceding the last delivered therapy and the 10 beats after this therapy. The print-out also shows the identity of the transmitting unit. In case of erroneous placement of the programmer head by the patient, an error message is transmitted in place of the usual print-out.

At St. George's Hospital, we started using this system over two years ago and it has remained in regular use despite the fact that, because it is a prototype, we have only been able to obtain four transmitter units. We were initially skeptical of its reliability and conducted a trial to confirm the repeatability of data transmission. Although some transmissions require more than one attempt to achieve a successful interrogation, we demonstrated 100% data concordance in 50 transmissions in which two complete interrogations were required.[5] Furthermore, in subsequent clinical use, we have never failed to obtain a successful transtelephonic interrogation from a patient. Because of our limited supply of transmitters, we issue them only to patients who are newly discharged from the hospital with a PCD™ implant or patients who are experiencing a period of relative instability in their arrhythmias. The transmitters are extremely popular with the patients and some difficulty has been experienced in persuading them to return them!

The Teletrace™ system clearly demonstrates the practicality of transtelephonic ICD interrogation and has proved a very useful tool in our follow-up clinic. The next generation of defibrillators offer even more programmable functions and greater storage of episode intervals and electrograms. However, as with the current generation of devices, these data will only be accessible when the patient visits the clinic, unless the challenge of producing a new range of transtelephonic data transmission systems is addressed.

Future Approaches to Transtelephonic Implantable Cardioverter-Defibrillator Monitoring

Data Transmission

The fundamental limitation governing such devices is that imposed by the telephone line itself. Although it allows simultaneous two-way communication, the data capacity of a conventional telephone line is limited. Additionally, regulations limit the types of apparatus that may be linked to the line and (in some countries) the type of information that may be transmitted over them. These regulations vary from country to country and this is one reason why Medtronic has not expanded the availability of the Teletrace™ ICD interrogation system that uses an acoustic coupler to send data in digital form. However, a number of "common currencies" exist on the international telephone system and these could be used to enable the development of a universal interrogation system.

For two-way communication, the digital (computer) modem offers a practical means of data transmission. With accepted international standards for this type of data transmission, a single device could be manufactured with a simple module connector to enable its use in any country. As many future ICD programmers are based around microcomputers, the incorporation of such a modem into the design would add little to the cost and dispense with the need for a dedicated transtelephonic receiver. Data compression techniques could be used to maximize the capacity of such a link.

An alternative approach for one-way communication would involve the incorporation of a facsimile modem in the patient unit. This would send the data received from interrogation of an ICD to any standard facsimile machine. This would again dispense with the need for a dedicated receiver and would enable an interrogation to be sent to a facsimile machine anywhere.

Practical Designs

While a number of transtelephonic monitoring systems could be designed, they fall into three main categories, as described below.

ICD memo

This would be a small, portable, battery-powered module capable of reading basic information about device status, programming, episode and therapy counts, last therapy details (probably intervals only), and a surface ECG rhythm strip. This information could be read into memory and then transmitted to the ICD clinic at the patient's convenience, either using an acoustic coupler or via a modem base station. Alternatively, the data could be stored on a magnetic medium (tape or disc) and mailed to the ICD clinic. Manufacture of such a system should be possible for a reasonable price and could be offered as an accessory to all patients or even included within the ICD price.

Programmable Interrogator

This would be a main-powered transportable unit linked directly to the patient's telephone line and would incorporate a telephone handset. For this device to be used, the patient would have to be in telephone contact with the ICD clinic. It would enable full interrogation of all device programming, datalogs, and stored electrograms, together with real-time electrogram and marker transmission. Duplex operation would enable the operator in the ICD clinic to select what information was transmitted to enable reduced transmission times. Such a "full-interrogation" system is likely to be considerably more expensive than the ICD memo and would probably be issued only to patients in whom there was concern over appropriate device function.

Full Transtelephonic Programmer

This device would again be a transportable base station but, in addition to the functions of the programmable interrogator, would allow limited programming changes to be made and pacing and sensing checks to be performed. While such devices could be used for individual patients, they might more appropriately be installed in "satellite clinics" established in areas in which a number of ICD patients live remotely from the main implanting center. Such a device is likely to be expensive and the market relatively small. Ideally, two telephone lines would be needed to allow simultaneous voice and data communication with the main ICD clinic.

Of these three devices, perhaps the ICD memo is the most attractive initially because of its low cost and the relatively simple technical problems involved in its design and certification. A full global market survey is probably needed to determine whether the potential demand for the more complex models described above justifies the effort involved in their development.

Conclusion

Transtelephonic monitoring of the ICD is a practical proposition and has a wide range of potential uses. The opportunity that it offers in improving the quality of life of ICD patients and in facilitating their follow-up has yet to be seized by ICD manufacturers. The potential role for transtelephonic programming is less clear, but in a limited form it could be of use. Whether the additional development costs and system complexity required to achieve safe transtelephonic ICD programming are indicated remains open to question.

References

1. Colbeck WJ, Hill DW, Mable SER, et al: Electrocardiographic transmissions by public telephone. Lancet 1968; 2:1017-1018.
2. Furman S, Parker B, Escher DJW: Transtelephone pacemaker clinic. J Thorac Cardiovasc Surg 1971; 61:827-834.
3. Dreifus LS, Zinberg A, Hurzeler P, et al: Transtelephonic monitoring of 25,919 implanted pacemakers. PACE 1986; 9:371-378.
4. Steinberg JS, Sugalaski JS: Cardiac rhythm precipitating automatic implantable-cardioverter defibrillator discharge in outpatient as detected from transtelephonic electrocardiographic recordings. Am J Cardiol 1991; 67:95-97.
5. Anderson MH, Paul VE, Jones S, et al: Transtelephonic interrogation of the implantable cardioverter defibrillator. PACE 1992; 15:1144-1150.

16

U-CARE:
Unexplained Cardiac Arrest Registry of Europe

S.G. Priori, on behalf of the Steering Committee of U-CARE:
M. Borggrefe, A.J. Camm, R.N.W. Hauer, H. Klein, K.-H. Kuck, P.J. Schwartz, P. Touboul, H.J.J. Wellens

Ventricular fibrillation (VF) in the setting of ischemic heart disease is the most widely recognized cause of sudden cardiac death. However, a wide range of less common causes is associated with VF such as cardiomyopathies, valvular defects, myocarditis, amyloidosis, hemochromatosis, and the long QT syndrome.

A minority of cases of VF occurs in patients in whom minimal or no cardiac abnormalities are identified in spite of an extensive cardiac evaluation. Some of these individuals die suddenly and even the postmortem examination cannot explain why VF had occurred.

The terms "idiopathic ventricular fibrillation" (IVF) or "primary electrical disease" have been used to identify this group of patients, but information presently available concerning this subgroup of patients experiencing cardiac arrest is scanty. For example, no accurate estimate of the incidence of IVF exists and it can only be inferred. It has been

From *Transvenous Defibrillation and Radiofrequency Ablation* edited by A. John Camm and Fred W. Lindemans © 1995, Futura Publishing Co., Inc., Armonk, NY.

reported that no cause is found in 1% of survivors of out-of-hospital cardiac arrest[1] and in 8% of patients dying suddenly.[2,3]

Assuming that this estimate is the most likely figure for the incidence of IVF, we should conclude that several thousands of individuals with a "normal" heart experience VF every year. At present, it is not known whether IVF is really "idiopathic" or if it is indeed an early symptom of a disease that will become fully manifest only years later. Even more puzzling questions concern the management of IVF patients, which is so far carried out on an empirical basis. It is not known whether these patients require therapy to prevent VF or if they are unlikely to experience recurrence even without intervention. The prognostic value of inducibility during electrical stimulation is not known and the importance of drug suppression of an inducible arrhythmia as a reliable index of effective treatment in this group of patients is unknown. Finally, the role of medical therapy versus no treatment or versus defibrillator implantation has still to be defined.

Current Knowledge about Idiopathic Ventricular Fibrillation

Only recently, a few groups[4-9] have started collecting data on small series of patients. We[10] reviewed studies published in the literature on the subject in the last 35 years: overall, 125 cases have been described. Complete information is, however, not available on the entire population. Sixty-eight percent of reported IVF occurred in men and 32% in women; the age range was 9 to 79 years; and the follow-up varied from 2 months to 14 years. Ninety-five patients underwent electrophysiological (EP) study and arrhythmias were induced in 55%: they ranged from couplets and triplets (7%) to nonsustained ventricular tachycardia (VT) (9%), sustained VT (26%), and VF (12%). Unfortunately, the number of monomorphic versus polymorphic VT cannot be obtained in a significant number of cases. The analysis of selected therapy in this group of patients is very complicated because virtually any intervention has been used: Class I antiarrhythmic agents, amiodarone, β-blockers, combinations of the above and, more recently, the implantable cardioverter-defibrillator (ICD). In order to evaluate if an interventional approach such as defibrillator implantation is worthwhile in patients with IVF, we should be able to have a reliable figure of the prognosis of these patients. Recently, Viskin and Belhassen[4] reported in their analysis of published cases of IVF a recurrence rate of 11% in 45 patients. In our analysis, with outcome data available for 100 patients, 12% of the patients died or had successful defibrillation by ICD. Additionally, another nine patients experienced recurrent nonsustained VT or syncopal episodes: the overall figure of patients with recurrent major cardiac arrhythmic events was 21%.[10] These data confirm the suggestions from the groups of Siebels et al[8] and Wever et al[9] that defibrillator implantation is warranted in IVF patients. However, to challenge this point of view, another study[6] has recently raised a word of caution. In this study, 25 ICDs were implanted in IVF patients and 13 discharges occurred, only two of which were appropriate and the remaining were related to physical exercise. In our analysis, 42 patients with ICDs were included and six appropriate shocks were delivered, most likely saving the lives of these six patients.

The conflicting reports on medical therapy and ICDs in this group of patients warrant a careful and controlled evaluation of their effectiveness as well as of their risks.

An extensive international data base of IVF is necessary in order to achieve a large, well-documented patient population from which not only epidemiologic figures of incidence and outcome can be derived but that can also serve for evaluation of the effectiveness of therapy in an homogeneous population. An additional advantage of an international data base is the possibility of spreading awareness among cardiologists about this under-recognized medical entity. For these reasons, the Unexplained Cardiac Arrest Registry of Europe (U-CARE) project was started under the umbrella of the Working Group on Cardiac Arrhythmias of the European Society of Cardiology.

Unexplained Cardiac Arrest Registry of Europe

U-CARE is the European project that will provide information on the incidence of IVF and will outline the profile of its victims. U-CARE is not a clinical trial; it is a registry open to anyone willing to participate. U-CARE provides no study protocol, but any physician is free to make his own judgments and he is only asked to report his decisions. One of the aims of the registry is, in fact, to evaluate what are the current therapeutic options selected by physicians to treat IVF.

Enrollment in the registry officially started January 1, 1993. So far, 37 patients have been enrolled: 27 in the retrospective section and 10 in the prospective section of the registry. The median age of patients is 32 years; 28 of the 37 (76%) are men and 9 of the 37 (24%) are women. The episode of VF occurred in 28 cases (76%) while the subjects were performing their everyday routine; in five cases (14%), exercise was associated with VF; in two cases (5%), intense emotions were associated with occurrence of VF; and finally, in the last two subjects (5%), VF occurred during sleep. Inducibility at EP study was observed in 14 of the 37 (38%) patients and the inducible rhythm was sustained VT in seven cases and VF in the remaining seven. It is interesting to observe that the predictive value of induction of VF at EP study is still controversial. While it was earlier suggested by Brugada et al[11] and by Morady and coworkers[12] that VF is a nonspecific response that can be induced even in normal hearts and has therefore no prognostic implications, more recently data obtained in the group of individuals resuscitated from out-of-hospital cardiac arrest[13] showed that induction of VF has the same prognostic value as VT. It will be interesting to evaluate the outcome of the seven patients enrolled in U-CARE with inducible VF. The analysis of the therapy selected by the physicians showed that, on the whole, all of the antiarrhythmic therapies have been used: 10 of the 37 (27%) patients received Class I agents; 4 of the 37 (11%) patients were treated with amiodarone; 6 of the 37 (16%) patients were treated with β-blockers; and 2 of the 37 (5%) patients were treated with calcium antagonists. Four of the 37 (11%) patients were not treated and all of them were reported by the same institution. Defibrillator implantation was selected as the most appropriate treatment for 15 of the 37 (41%) patients and it was, therefore, the treatment of choice in most cases. It is interesting to observe that the patients who received, alone or in combination, a Class I agent were treated before 1988. Since then, no Class I drug was prescribed. On the other hand, most ICDs were implanted after 1988, suggesting a change in the attitude of physicians who were probably influenced by the "post-CAST effect" on one side and reassured by the improved technology of the ICD on the other.

Recurrence of VF can be estimated so far only from the data of the 27 patients of the retrospective portion of the study. The follow-up of this group of patients ranged between 1 and 10 years and no patient was diagnosed with cardiac disease. Ventricular fibrillation recurred in 6 of the 27 (22%) patients, thus confirming the rather high risk of a second cardiac arrest in this group of patients, as has recently been suggested by Siebels et al[8] and Wever et al[9] Two patients experienced recurrence after an ICD was implanted and they were successfully resuscitated; three patients received therapy with Class I agents; and one was treated with amiodarone. No inappropriate discharges of the ICD were reported in the 15 patients who were implanted, suggesting that data reported by Meissner et al[6] may no longer apply to the most recent generation of ICDs.

The Future of U-CARE

Since the start of U-CARE, some important findings such as the high risk of recurrence of an episode of cardiac arrest in this group of patients have already been highlighted. Although more data are required to reach conclusive statements, the fact that no patient from the retrospective branch of the study developed overt cardiac disease suggests that a primary electrical disease may indeed occur in otherwise normal hearts. If the enrollment of U-CARE continues at the present rate, it will be possible to provide more detailed guidelines for the treatment of IVF patients in the near future. Additionally, U-CARE will be an important tool to raise the awareness of physicians about the existence of such a neglected disease and will foster cooperation to disclose the many unknown aspects of IVF.

References

1. Myerburg RJ, Conde CA, Sung RJ, et al: Clinical, electrophysiologic and hemodynamic profile of patients resuscitated from pre-hospital cardiac arrest. Am J Med 1980; 68:568-576.
2. Friedman M, Manwaring JH, Rosemann RH, et al: Instantaneous and sudden deaths. JAMA 1973; 225:1319-1328.
3. Raymand JR, Van der Berg EK Jr, Knapp MJ: Non-traumatic pre-hospital sudden death in young adults. Arch Intern Med 1988; 148:303-308.
4. Viskin S, Belhassen B: Idiopathic ventricular fibrillation. Am Heart J 1990; 120:661-671.
5. Martini B, Nava A, Thiene G, et al: Ventricular fibrillation without apparent heart disease: Description of six cases. Am Heart J 1989; 118:1203-1209.
6. Meissner RD, Mosteller RT, Steinman M, et al: Cardiac arrest in patients without significant structural heart disease: A multicenter experience with implantable cardioverter defibrillator therapy. J Am Coll Cardiol 1991; 17:92A.
7. Wellens HJJ, Lemery R, Smith JL, et al: Sudden arrhythmic death without overt heart disease. Circulation 1992; 85(I):192-197.
8. Siebels J, Schneider MAE, Geiger M, et al: Unexpected recurrences in survivors of cardiac arrest without organic heart disease. Eur Heart J 1991; 12:535. Abstract.
9. Wever E, Hauer R, Oomen P, et al: Unfavorable outcome in patients with primary electrical disease who survived unexpected cardiac arrest. Eur Heart J 1991; 12:534. Abstract.
10. Priori SG, Borggrefe M, Camm AJ, et al: Unexplained cardiac arrest. The need for a prospective registry. Eur Heart J 1992; 13:1445-1446.
11. Brugada P, Green M, Abdollah H, et al: Significance of ventricular arrhythmias initiated by programmed electrical stimulation: The importance of the type of ventricular arrhythmia induced and the number of premature stimuli required. Circulation 1984; 69:87-92.

12. Morady F, Shapiro W, Shen E, et al: Programmed ventricular stimulation in patients without spontaneous ventricular tachycardia. Am Heart J 1984; 107:875-882.
13. Poole JE, Mathisen TL, Kudenchuk PJ, et al: Long-term outcome in patients who survive out of hospital ventricular fibrillation and undergo electrophysiologic studies: Evaluation by electrophysiologic subgroups. J Am Coll Cardiol 1990; 16:657-665.

17
Defibrillator Implantation for Patients with Primary Electrical Disease

R.N.W. Hauer

Several reports have shown an excellent prognosis for patients with ventricular tachyarrhythmias who have no evidence of structural heart disease. Prognosis may be worse, however, in the subgroup of these patients with primary electrical disease who experienced a cardiac arrest episode.

This chapter evaluates the outcome in a group of patients with primary electrical disease who survived a cardiac arrest due to either ventricular fibrillation (VF) or rapid ventricular tachycardia (VT). The role that the implantable cardioverter-defibrillator (ICD) may play in these patients is also discussed. The data have been collected as part of a prospective study in the University Hospital in Utrecht, The Netherlands, which started in 1984 and lasted until 1991.

Diagnostic Procedures

The diagnosis of primary electrical disease was made after careful cardiological examination including two-dimensional and Doppler echocardiography, nuclear scintigraphy, left and right heart catheterization with cineangiography, and right ventricular biopsies at multiple

From *Transvenous Defibrillation and Radiofrequency Ablation* edited by A. John Camm and Fred W. Lindemans © 1995, Futura Publishing Co., Inc., Armonk, NY.

sites. Persistent or transient long QT syndrome as well as preexcitation were excluded.

Patient Population

There were 17 males (74%) and 6 females with a mean age of 32 years (range 13 to 66 years) in the study. The presenting arrhythmia was VF in 17 patients (74%) and VT with loss of consciousness in 6 (26%), of whom 5 had required cardiopulmonary resuscitation. The arrhythmia was exercise related in six patients.

Although there was no evidence of structural heart disease in any of these patients, nine (39%) showed abnormalities in the electrocardiogram (ECG). Most of these were minor and nonspecific: abnormal repolarization in seven, abnormal intraventricular conduction in six, high voltage in V_5 and V_6 without other signs of left ventricular hypertrophy in two, low voltage ECG in one, and atrial fibrillation in one.

Programmed Stimulation

Programmed electrical stimulation was performed in the right ventricular apex and in the right ventricular outflow tract with up to three extrastimuli at basic cycle lengths of 600 and 430 milliseconds and included long-short cycles. In patients who were not inducible, the protocol was repeated during isoproterenol infusion.

In five patients (22%), rapid monomorphic VT could be induced. In 10 (43%), the induced arrhythmia was polymorphic VT or VF. No significant ventricular tachyarrhythmia could be induced in eight patients (35%).

Therapy at Discharge

At discharge, 10 patients were treated with antiarrhythmic drugs, guided by the findings of continuous telemetry, Holter recordings, exercise testing, and the electrophysiological (EP) study. After failure of drug treatment, two patients received map-guided cryosurgery and one received catheter ablation. Ten patients received an ICD; six of them because of baseline noninducibility, which prevented therapy assessment, and four of them because antiarrhythmic drug therapy failed.

Follow-up Results

During an average follow-up of 38 months (range 5 to 85 months), seven patients (30%) experienced a major arrhythmic event. Two of them died suddenly out-of-hospital, one was resuscitated after recurrent VF, and four showed a (pre)syncopal episode terminated by ICD shock. Termination of a rapid ventricular tachyarrhythmia by a shock from the ICD was documented on Holter in one of these four patients. Therefore, convincing evidence of the life-threatening nature of the arrhythmic event was obtained in four of the seven patients with major arrhythmia recurrence, representing 17% of the total group. None of the patients with an ICD died or required resuscitation.

The first of the two patients who died suddenly had been on quinidine therapy for three years. Ventricular fibrillation had been induced at his baseline EP study with two extrastimuli. The second patient, who had monomorphic VT induced at baseline EP study, died suddenly about half a year after cryosurgery.

The third patient, with VF induced at the baseline study, was resuscitated successfully from VF, after having been on flecainide for about two years. Of the four patients receiving shocks from the ICD, one had polymorphic VT induced at baseline and three were noninducible.

Conclusions

1. Cardiac arrest in patients with primary electrical disease is associated with a high incidence of life-threatening arrhythmic events during long-term follow-up.
2. Implantable cardioverter-defibrillator implantation should be considered as a therapy of first choice, especially in patients without reliable indicators for guiding therapy.
3. Noninducibility during programmed electrical stimulation does not identify a subgroup with a favorable outcome.

Especially in these patients, where knowledge about the mechanisms of ventricular tachyarrhythmias is lacking, the ICD should provide extensive monitoring capabilities of the electrogram prior to and after therapy delivery.

18

MIRRACLEs: A Study of Prevention of Sudden Cardiac Death in High-Risk Patients by Defibrillator Implantation Early after Acute Myocardial Infarction

L. Jordaens

Sudden cardiac death (in most instances due to ventricular tachyarrhythmias) remains the most important cause of death after survival of the acute phase of myocardial infarction (MI).[1,2] Even with modern treatment including thrombolytics, aspirin, β-blockers, and angiotensin converting enzyme (ACE) inhibitors, the sudden death rate remains about 5% over a follow-up of one year.[3,4] It is clear that antiarrhythmic drugs do not improve survival, as has been shown by the Cardiac Arrhythmia Suppression Trial (CAST) study, even when they are used to reduce spontaneous asymptomatic ventricular arrhythmias.[5] Recent small trials with amiodarone showed a tendency to reduce the sudden death rate.[6] However, it is clear that amiodarone is associated with severe side effects and that many patients cannot be treated on a long-term basis with such a drug.[7] The European Myocardial Infarct Amiodarone Trial (EMIAT) is ongoing and the recruiting phase will probably

From *Transvenous Defibrillation and Radiofrequency Ablation* edited by A. John Camm and Fred W. Lindemans © 1995, Futura Publishing Co., Inc., Armonk, NY.

end in 1994. Studies with β-blockers and the recent studies with amiodarone were undertaken in large cohorts of patients, without attempts to stratify these groups into subgroups with an increased risk for sudden death. For example, EMIAT uses only a low left ventricular ejection fraction (LVEF) as a criterion for inclusion and does not take markers for electrical risk into account. However, very high-risk patients for sudden death after infarction can now be recognized, with a risk up to 35% in some subgroups.[4,8,9] Such a sudden death rate is higher than that of patients with ventricular tachycardia (VT) who receive therapy guided by Holter or programmed electrical stimulation. This implies that it could even be considered unethical to withhold a therapy that is effective in preventing sudden death in such patients.

Intervention with an antiarrhythmic device (an implantable cardioverter-defibrillator [ICD]) is tempting because of its proven efficacy in survivors of sudden death. Many preliminary ideas on the topic of preventive implantation have been published in the recent past.[10,11] However, the costs are high and the technology is not yet perfect.

Furthermore, in spite of an increasing knowledge about the arrhythmic substrate, the spontaneous triggers of life-threatening arrhythmias, and the importance of the autonomic nervous system, stratification of patients surviving MI into high-risk groups for sudden (and total cardiac) death remains difficult.

Therefore, we propose "MIRRACLEs." The acronym MIRRACLEs stands for "Myocardial Infarction Risk Recognition And Conversion of Life-threatening Events (into survival)." From its name, it is clear that such study includes a stratification and an intervention branch. The latter will be focused on safety and efficacy of ICD implantation in very high-risk groups that have been defined in earlier studies.

Most details discussed below concern the intervention branch since its organization took the most time and because its concept made the stratification branch possible. Many details in the stratification study still have to be discussed, but data sampling has already begun in two hospitals.

Aim of the Study

The aim of a study with an intervention should be to reduce sudden death by at least 80% to 90% in a high-risk group that needs to be defined and to reduce total mortality in this high-risk group as well. It would be very good if the cardiac death rate could be reduced by this intervention in the total study group as well (i.e., in the total group from which the study patients were recruited). This would make such an approach acceptable from a socioeconomic point of view. It is clear that a very large recruitment area will be needed to find patients who are suitable for therapy with a device.

In the stratification branch, the definition of "high risk" has to be refined. In this preliminary phase, data will be collected in parallel with the intervention branch and in more centers to enhance future integration with other projects (as pointed out with the European Working Group on Arrhythmias). Therefore, all available data (clinical, electrocardiographic) will be stored. Part of these data will be analyzed prospectively to assess the value of this information with respect to prognosis, and part will be kept on optical disk for later retrieval when more advanced software is available.

In this phase, the intervention study should be a feasibility and safety study in which attention will be paid in particular to safety and complications associated with the procedure in the first six weeks after implantation. Late follow-up would focus on endpoints as summarized in the later sections (mortality, arrhythmias).

Statistical Requirements

It is anticipated that at least 500 patients will have to be screened in order to find a subgroup that is acceptable for this kind of intervention. By selecting about 20 patients from this total group to constitute the high-risk group, implantation of an ICD would reduce sudden death in this subgroup not from 35% to 0% but from 35% to 17.5%, because a control group is included. This means that 3.5 lives would be saved and that 6.5 devices should be considered as being wasted in the first year of follow-up. This remains comparable with the use of ICDs in survivors of ventricular fibrillation (VF).

The impact of this intervention on overall survival would be an improvement of 0.7% for the total group of 500 patients. This could become 1.4% if the control group were also treated with an ICD. These data correspond with figures obtained from a Belgian pilot study and are a pessimistic view.[8]

Specific Goal of a Pilot Intervention Study

It is not unthinkable that implantation of an ICD early after infarction will be associated with particular problems. For instance, implantation in a diseased right ventricle early after infarction could result in perforation, pericardial effusion, tamponade, or could be associated with a poor quality of the electrical signal. Undersensing after a shock could happen in such a situation. Arrhythmic storms in the early phase after an acute MI can also occur. These are arguments to randomize patients who are judged as bearing a high risk and to take the chance that they will not receive active treatment.

Practical Considerations of Organization

Each intervention center should create a data base of infarctions and have regional cardiological centers contribute to this data base. A coordinating center should randomize patients to active or control therapy. The intervention center could implant the ICD. Follow-up can be performed in the regional center.

Since a grant was obtained from the National Fund for Scientific Research (NFWO), a pilot study to examine the feasibility of a larger project will be conducted in Ghent, Belgium. Approval of the Ethics Committee of the NFWO was obtained in 1991 before submission of the project to the NFWO.

Inclusion and Exclusion Criteria

It is clear that patients should be studied early after infarction since the highest mortality is observed within the first few months after MI. Infarction should be transmural, following classical World Health Organization criteria. All patients should receive standard therapy, including aspirin, β-blockers, if possible, and ACE inhibitors with a short half-life, according to the Survival And Ventricular Enlargement (SAVE) protocol. Diuretics should be avoided.[12]

The most important measurement to be done between day 7 and day 12 is determination of LVEF (with radionuclides to avoid measurement errors between individual centers). A cutoff point at 35% will be used as this seems to be compatible with most ongoing studies. If LVEF <35% is associated with one of the following, a patient can be included in the *intervention arm*:

- presence of late potentials (40 Hz filter, <1 μV noise, filtered QRS duration >110 milliseconds with low amplitude signal >40 milliseconds)

- transient or permanent bundle branch block after the infarction
- reduced heart rate variability (standard deviation [SDNN] <50 milliseconds on 24-hour heart rate)

In patients who are eligible for intervention and are in the *stratification* groups, further data are stored concerning autonomic function (baroreflex sensitivity), the presence of spontaneous ventricular premature beats, and the presence of abnormalities in the behavior of the QT interval.[13-15]

A patient will be excluded from the intervention arm if his general condition does not permit inclusion (for example, neuropsychiatric disease, malignancy, severe cerebrovascular disease). Another important exclusion is the presence of unstable angina and New York Heart Association functional Class IV. No antiarrhythmic drugs are acceptable except digoxin. See Figure 1 for a schematic outline of the inclusion criteria.

Choice of the Device

The device should be able to provide bradycardia backup pacing (40 to 45 beats/min) and shocks for VF. Antitachycardia pacing should not be a requirement in this phase of the study. Information storage on the arrhythmia that has been treated is necessary.[16]

Randomization and Procedure

High-risk patients in intervention centers are randomized to intervention or control. All will receive an ACE inhibitor according to SAVE guidelines. Intervention will imply implantation of an ICD with transvenous leads. Three consecutive successful conversions of VF or ventricular flutter at a 24 J level must be documented. The configuration should be adapted to the status of the patient. Before discharge, a checkup should be performed including a noninvasive electrophysiological study. The group that is assigned to control should receive follow-up at the same rate as the active arm. Regular Holter recordings should be performed to assure comparable intensity of follow-up.

Endpoints

The primary endpoint in the intervention arm is death from all causes. This should be further classified as sudden cardiac death, total

Inclusion Criteria

Q-wave Infarction
(criteria W.H.O.)

Standard therapy
(ASA/Betablockers/ACE inhibitors)

day 7-12

EF < 0.35

and

BRS ↓
QTc ↑

LP +

BBB
transient /
permanent

HRV ↓

randomization

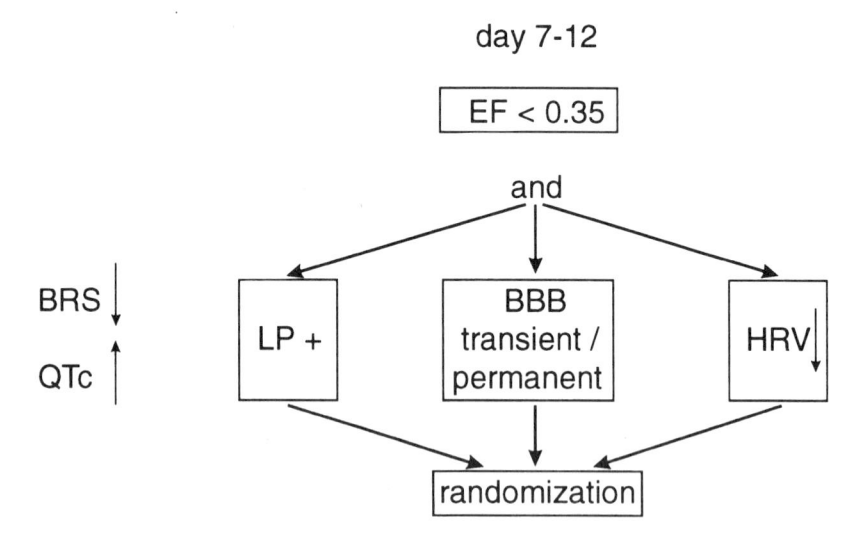

Figure 1. *Summary of the inclusion criteria for the intervention arm of the study. ASA: acetylsalicylic acid; EF: ejection fraction; BRS: baroreflex sensitivity; QTc: corrected QT interval; LP: late potentials; BBB: bundle branch block; HRV: heart rate variability.*

cardiac death, and death from other causes. Other important secondary endpoints are the presence of sustained VT and the occurrence of aborted sudden death due to VF that was terminated by a successful resuscitation. Interrogation of the implanted device should be an additional helpful diagnostic tool in the evaluation of the treatment. In the stratification arm, follow-up will be performed at one and two years, with direct mailing to general practitioners and with a check on mortality data in the official files of the government.

Conclusions

Even if intervention for larger groups will not be miraculous, it could be highly desirable for some patients to receive an ICD. If the safety of such a procedure could be established in this study, its principal goal will be reached. Furthermore, a local network of centers showing interest for such prospective work would be established, thereby helping to redefine criteria for high risk in a larger European context.

References

1. Moss AJ, Benhorin J: Prognosis and management after a first myocardial infarction. N Engl J Med 1990; 322:743-753.
2. Multicenter Postinfarction Research Group: Risk stratification and survival after myocardial infarction. N Engl J Med 1983; 309:331.
3. Pfeffer MA, Braunwald E, Moyé LA, et al on behalf of the SAVE Investigators: Effect of captopril on mortality and morbidity in patients with left ventricular dysfunction after myocardial infarction. N Engl J Med 1992; 327:669-677.
4. Jordaens L, Schoenfeld Ph, Block P, et al: Risk stratification after infarction: Final results of a multicenter prospective study. Circulation 1991; 84(II):238. Abstract.
5. The Cardiac Arrhythmia Suppression Trial (CAST): Preliminary report: Effect of encainide and flecainide on mortality in a randomized trial of arrhythmia suppression after myocardial infarction. N Engl J Med 1989; 321:406.
6. Ceremuzynski L, Kleczar E, Krzeminska-Pakula M, et al: Effect of amiodarone on mortality after myocardial infarction: A double-blind, placebo-controlled, pilot study. J Am Coll Cardiol 1992; 20:1056-1062.
7. Koonlawee N: The Amiodarone odyssey. J Am Coll Cardiol 1992; 20:1063-1065.
8. Jordaens L, Schoenfeld Ph, Demeester C, et al: Late potentials and ejection fraction at hospital discharge: Prognostic value in thrombolyzed and non-thrombolyzed patients. Acta Cardiologica 1991; XLVI:531-541.
9. Cripps T, Bennett ED, Camm AJ, et al: High gain signal averaged electrocardiogram combined with 24 hour monitoring in patients early after myocardial infarction for bedside prediction of arrhythmic events. Br Heart J 1988; 60:181-187.
10. Anderson MH, Camm AJ: Implications for present and future applications of the implantable cardioverter-defibrillator resulting from the use of a simple model of cost efficacy. Br Heart J 1993; 69:83-92.
11. Farrel TG, Bashir Y, Cripps T, et al: Risk stratification for arrhythmic events in postinfarction patients based on heart rate variability, ambulatory electrocardiographic variables and the signal-averaged electrocardiogram. J Am Coll Cardiol 1991; 18:687-697.
12. Olsson G, Rydén L: Prevention of sudden death using β-blockers. Circulation 1991; 84(VI):33-37.
13. La Rovere MT, Specchia G, Mortara A, et al: Baroreflex sensitivity, clinical correlates, and cardiovascular mortality among patients with a first myocardial infarction. A prospective study. Circulation 1988; 78:816-824.
14. Day CP, McComb JM, Campbell RWF: QT dispersion: An indication of arrhythmia risk in patients with long QT intervals. Br Heart J 1990; 63:342.

15. Lombardi F, Sandrone G, Mortara A, et al: Circadian variation of spectral indices of heart rate variability after myocardial infarction. Am Heart J 1992; 123:1521-1529.
16. Fromer M, Brachmann J, Block M, et al: Efficacy of automatic multimodal device therapy for ventricular tachyarrhythmias as delivered by a new implantable pacing cardioverter-defibrillator: Results of a European Multicenter Study of 102 implants. Circulation 1992; 86:363-374.

19

The Future of Arrhythmia Surgery

O.C.K.M. Penn

Surgery for cardiac arrhythmias became possible with the development of methods to induce and localize tachycardia in the human heart; i.e., the technique of programmed electrical stimulation first applied by Wellens, Durrer, and Coumel about 25 years ago.[1,2]

Surgery for cardiac arrhythmias requires close cooperation and mutual understanding between the surgeon and the clinical electrophysiologist.

The basic approach in surgical treatment of cardiac arrhythmias is the following:

1. identify the mechanism of the cardiac arrhythmia;
2. localize the site of origin or the vulnerable portion of the arrhythmia pathway; and
3. ablate the site of origin or part of the arrhythmia pathway.

The ideal technique for surgical treatment of cardiac arrhythmias

1. preserves the structural integrity of the tissue;
2. has minimal effect on normal structure and function;
3. creates a nonarrhythmogenic, homogeneous lesion;
4. may be performed in a reversible manner;
5. allows continuous assessment; and
6. can be employed rapidly.

From *Transvenous Defibrillation and Radiofrequency Ablation* edited by A. John Camm and Fred W. Lindemans © 1995, Futura Publishing Co., Inc., Armonk, NY.

178 • TRANSVENOUS DEFIBRILLATION AND RF ABLATION

Radiofrequency (RF) ablation with a catheter also meets most of these requirements.

With the direct surgical approach of cardiac arrhythmias, attempts are made to divide, remove, interrupt, and destruct accessory pathways, areas of reentry, or areas of abnormal automaticity.

With the indirect approach, the milieu of the substrate is modified, propagation of the arrhythmia is prevented, or pacing or defibrillation devices are implanted for termination of arrhythmias.

The indications for arrhythmia surgery are inefficacy of antiarrhythmic drug therapy, noncompliance with prescribed drug treatment, side effects of antiarrhythmic drugs, or failure of catheter ablation attempts.

Figure 1 shows a cost projection for medical and surgical treatment of arrhythmias in patients with the Wolff-Parkinson-White (WPW) syndrome. The initial costs of surgical treatment are relatively high, but the ongoing expenses of medical treatment, including the need for re-hospitalizations, are reaching the same level after about 12 years. Although this has not been analyzed yet, catheter ablation may well provide a more favorable cost picture.

Figure 2 illustrates the various tachycardia mechanisms that can be treated with surgery, as follows:

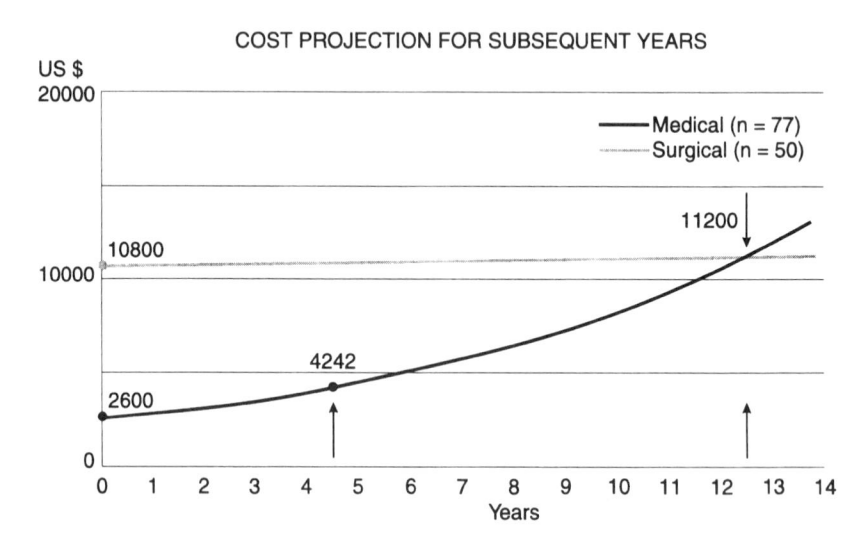

Figure 1. *Comparison of projected costs for surgical and medical treatment of tachyarrhythmias based on 77 WPW patients treated with antiarrhythmic drugs during 4.5 years and 50 WPW patients receiving arrhythmia surgery.*

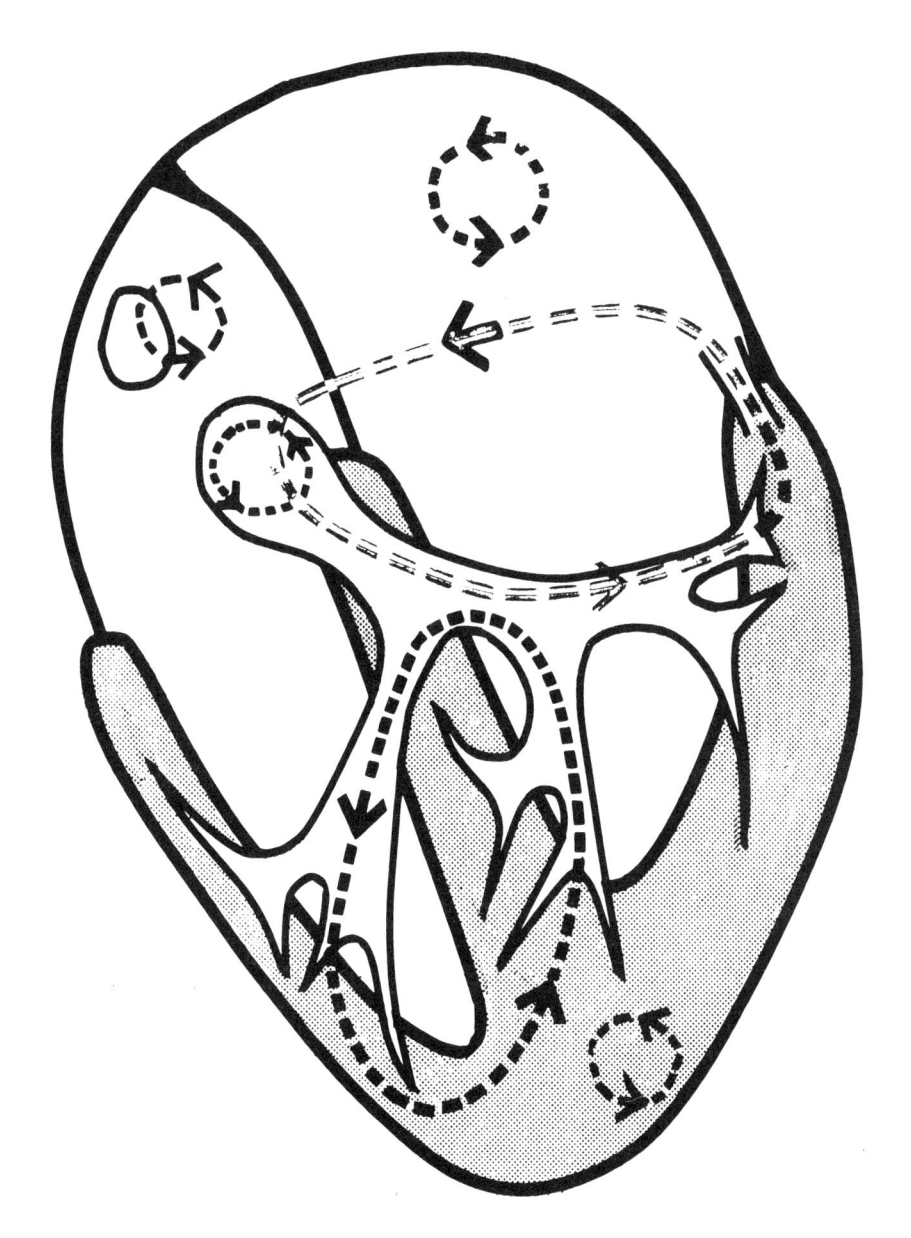

Figure 2. *Schematic representation of tachycardia mechanisms that can be treated surgically. Courtesy of H.J.J. Wellens.*

atrial tachycardia;

atrioventricular (AV) nodal tachycardia;

accessory pathway-based reentry tachycardia; and

ventricular tachycardia (VT).

Atrial Tachycardia

In atrial tachycardia, the site of abnormal impulse formation is identified by mapping the activation of the atrium using a spoon electrode with 250 electrodes as it was developed by Allessie. The abnormal area is then isolated or removed by means of cryoablation. Radiofrequency ablation does not, yet, provide a suitable alternative for the surgical approach for this type of patient.

Atrial Flutter and Fibrillation

Surgical techniques for the treatment of atrial flutter or atrial fibrillation (AF), aiming at either interruption of the reentry circuit or isolation or removal of the area of abnormal impulse formation, are currently under study. Guiraudon et al[3] developed the atrial corridor operation. With this technique, a single isolated corridor for activation propagation from the sinus node to the entry of the AV node is created. It is important to isolate the right and the left atrium from the ventricles, always cryoablating the area underneath the coronary sinus, in order not to leave any conducting fibers to the ventricles.

Cox et al[4] developed the maze operation for AF, of which already some modifications exist. With this approach, several incisions are made in the atria with the purpose of confining atrial activation to limited and predefined pathways, while blocking potential routes for macro reentry. The long-term success rate of this approach, however, is still unclear at this moment.

The problem of thrombus formation and subsequent embolization in AF has remained unsolved so far.

Atrioventricular Nodal Tachycardia

Two techniques are used for the surgical treatment of AV nodal tachycardia in which extranodal pathways provide one limb of the reentry circuit:

1. incision in the retrograde limb of the circuit[5] and
2. cryoablation of a large part of the atrial input into the AV node.[6]

We have mainly used the second technique, applying cryoablation at multiple sites at the atrial input of the AV node in the region between the coronary sinus, the ring of the tricuspid valve, and the tendon of Todaro.

Wolff-Parkinson-White Tachycardia

Tachycardias in the WPW syndrome are circus movement tachycardias with an accessory AV pathway incorporated in the circuit. A short antegrade refractory period of the accessory pathway poses significant risk to these patients in case of AF.

Before the widespread use of RF ablation, surgical treatment of the WPW syndrome was considered:

1. **strictly indicated** in case of severe symptoms (syncope) or failure of medical treatment;
2. **indicated** in any patient requiring treatment if the patient or the physician preferred the surgical approach;
3. **not indicated** in asymptomatic preexcitation; and
4. **contraindicated** in patients with associated cardiac or extracardiac conditions with a fatal short-term outcome or markedly increased surgical risk.

Today, failure of catheter ablation is the only indication for surgery for the WPW syndrome.

There are two surgical techniques for the WPW syndrome:

1. endocardial dissection and interruption of the accessory pathway using cardioplegic arrest[7] and
2. epicardial dissection and cryoablation of the accessory pathway in a beating heart.[8]

Figure 3 illustrates the number of WPW operations per year that were performed in Maastricht, The Netherlands, showing a sharp decline with the introduction of RF catheter ablation.

Ventricular Tachycardia

In The Netherlands, with a population of almost 15 million people, ventricular arrhythmias and pump failure each claim slightly over

WPW per year
sept 1986 - aug 1991

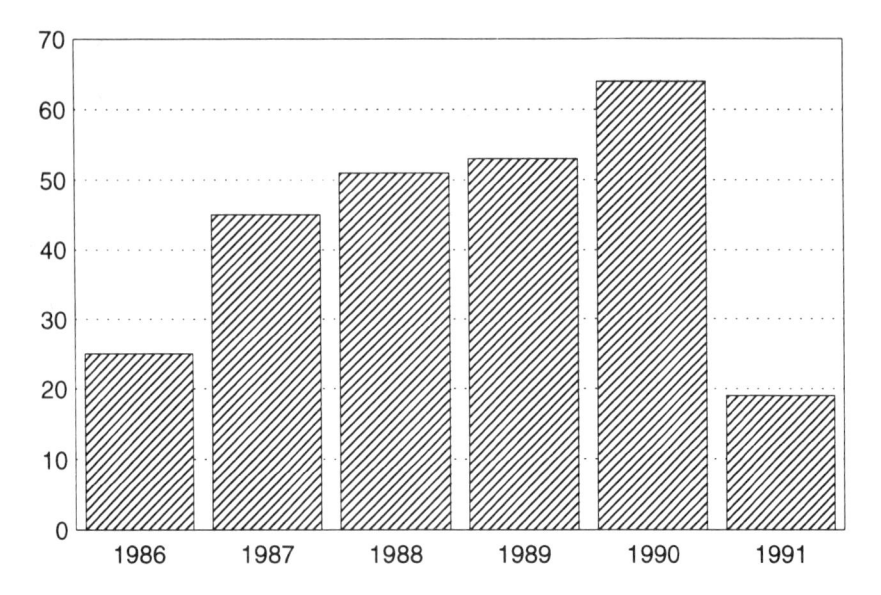

Figure 3. *Number of WPW operations per year in Maastricht, The Netherlands.*

10,000 deaths per year. Both causes of death have shown a gradual increase over the last decade, contrasting sharply with a decrease in ischemia-related death from about 47,000 per year in 1980 to about 40,000 per year in 1990. If these trends are linearly extrapolated, each of these three causes of death would claim about 20,000 victims by the year 2010.

The surgical technique for VT depends on the etiology and the location of the VT. The majority of procedures is performed in patients who suffered a myocardial infarction (MI). Other pathologies leading to VT that may be treated with surgery are arrhythmogenic right ventricular dysplasia, correction of tetralogy of Fallot, ventricular tumor, ventricular trauma, and mitral valve prolapse. The natural history of ventricular tachyarrhythmias in the University Hospital in Maastricht are listed in Table 1. It is clear that the sudden death rate and the late mortality are very different for the five indications listed.

Four surgical techniques have been developed to prevent conduction to and from the arrhythmogenic substrate in the ventricle:

Table 1
Mortality for Ventricular Tachycardia at the University Hospital in Maastricht, The Netherlands

Arrhythmia	Number of Patients	Follow-up (Months)	Sudden Death Rate	Mortality Rate
ARVD	11	39	0%	19%
Idiopathic VT	52	86	0%	2%
Idiopathic VF	6	39	0%	0%
Postinfarction VT	79	26	6%	19%
Postinfarction VF	37	22	14%	35%

ARVD: arrhythmogenic right ventricular dysplasia; VT: ventricular tachycardia; VF: ventricular fibrillation.

1. incision or right ventricular disconnection in case of arrhythmogenic right ventricular dysplasia, which has almost completely been abandoned now;
2. encircling endocardial ventriculotomy around the border zone of the infarcted tissue, developed by Guiraudon,[9] that is considered to be slightly more damaging to the ventricle than
3. endocardial resection for VT after MI, developed by Josephson et al,[10] that is commonly practiced in our hospital; and
4. cryoablation, which is commonly combined with endocardial resection after MI but which is rarely performed for idiopathic VT nowadays.

Figure 4 illustrates the techniques of aneurysmectomy, endocardial excision, and encircling ventriculotomy.

Ventricular Fibrillation

A direct surgical treatment for ventricular fibrillation (VF) is impossible because of the inability to localize a site of origin. Therefore, the approach of implanting an automatic defibrillator is preferred.

Conclusions

Based on the experience in our center, the expected need for the various procedures in the Netherlands is listed in Table 2. It shows

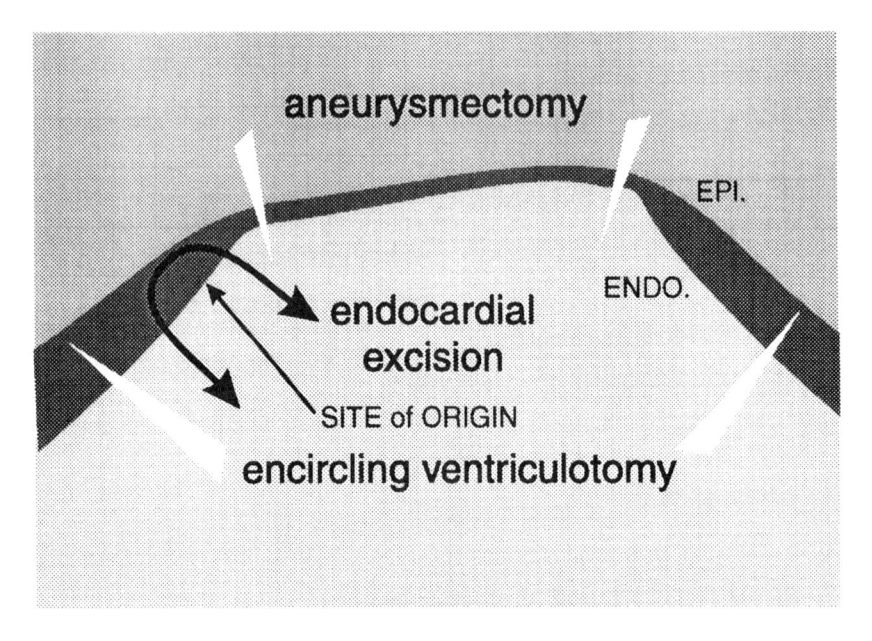

Figure 4. *Schematic illustration of aneurysmectomy, encircling ventriculotomy, and endocardial excision (resection).*

Table 2
Expected Need for Surgical Interventions for Cardiac Arrhythmias in The Netherlands

Arrhythmia	RF Ablation	Surgery	ICD
WPW	575	40	—
AV nodal	250	—	—
AF	100	?	—
VT	—	40	—
VF	—	—	150

RF: radiofrequency; ICD: implantable cardioverter-defibrillator; WPW: Wolff-Parkinson-White; AV: atrioventricular; AF: atrial fibrillation; VT: ventricular tachycardia; VF: ventricular fibrillation.

that RF ablation will be applied in the majority of cases of WPW tachycardia, AV nodal tachycardia, and AF/atrial flutter.

Surgical therapy will probably be limited to a small percentage of WPW patients, a minority of VT patients, and an as yet unknown number of patients with AF/atrial flutter. We expect that the implantable cardioverter-defibrillator will mainly be applied in patients resuscitated from VF.

Acknowledgments: I gratefully acknowledge the help and inspiration of my colleague Hein Wellens.

References

1. Durrer D, Schoo L, Schuilenburg RM, et al: The role of premature beats in the initiation and the termination of supraventricular tachycardia in the Wolff-Parkinson-White syndrome. Circulation 1967; 36:644.
2. Coumel Ph, Cabrol P, Fabiato A, et al: Tachycardie permanente par rythme reciproque. 1.Preuves du diagnostic par stimulation auriculaire et ventriculaire. Arch Mal Coeur 1967; 60:1830.
3. Guiraudon GM, Campbell CS, Jones DL, et al: Combined sinoatrial node atrioventricular isolation: A surgical alternative to His bundle ablation in patients with atrial fibrillation. Circulation 1985; II75(4):III-220. Abstract.
4. Cox JL, Schuessler RB, Cain ME, et al: Surgery for atrial fibrillation. Sem Thorac Cardiovasc Surg 1989; 1(1):67.
5. Johnson DC, Nunn GR, Richards DA, et al: Surgical therapy for supraventricular tachycardia, a potentially curable disorder. J Thorac Cardiovasc Surg 1987; 93:913.
6. Cox JL, Holman WL, Cain ME, et al: Cryosurgical treatment of atrioventricular node reentrant tachycardia. Circulation 1987; 76:1329.
7. Sealy WC, Gallagher JJ, Wallace AG: The surgical treatment of Wolff-Parkinson-White Syndrome: Evaluation of improved methods for identification and interruption of the Kent Bundle. Ann Thorac Surg 1976; 22(5):443.
8. Guiraudon GM, Klein GJ, Gulamhusein S, et al: Surgical repair of Wolff-Parkinson-White syndrome: A new closed-heart technique. Ann Thorac Surg 1984; 37(1):67.
9. Guiraudon GM, Fontaine G, Frank R, et al: Encircling endocardial ventriculotomy: A new surgical treatment for life-threatening ventricular tachycardias resistant to medical treatment following myocardial infarction. Ann Thorac Surg 1978; 26:438.
10. Josephson ME, Harken AH, Horowitz LN, et al: Endocardial excision: A new surgical technique for the treatment of recurrent ventricular tachycardia. Circulation 1979; 60:1430.

20

Principles and Techniques of Catheter Ablation

E. Rowland, A.D. Cunningham

Cardiac ablation is the application of energy or substances to the heart with the purpose of modifying or preventing local activation through the controlled destruction or modification of cells.

Many different methods have been developed and tested to damage myocardial cells in a controllable and useful way by using a catheter to reach the target area. The suggested methods of catheter ablation have been:

1. application of an electrical impulse of very high energy content, a technique used in one of the earliest animal studies of electrical ablation and in which shocks of 500 J from a defibrillator were delivered via a half-shell electrode[1];
2. application of an electrical impulse of high energy (50 to 360 J), using a standard defibrillator and standard pacing catheters[2];
3. application of low levels of electrical energy (2 to 40 J), using a discharging capacitor (low energy ablator) and an electrode with large surface area and modified geometry[3];
4. application of alternating current in the radiofrequency (RF) range using a standard electrode[4] or an electrode with large surface area[5];

From *Transvenous Defibrillation and Radiofrequency Ablation* edited by A. John Camm and Fred W. Lindemans © 1995, Futura Publishing Co., Inc., Armonk, NY.

5. transcoronary infusion, after selective coronary cannulation, of ethanol[6] or collagen[7] for ablation or modification of ventricular myocardium or atrioventricular (AV) nodal conduction;
6. application of a thermal induction loop[8];
7. local "freezing" of tissue using a cryothermal catheter[9]; and
8. application of microwave radiation with a "wave guide" catheter and adjustable antenna.[10]

The energy source used for ablation is only one part of the system and specialized catheters are often required to apply the energy to the tissue in a safe and effective way.

Some of the techniques listed above have not (yet) been developed into clinical practice, while the most successfully applied approaches have all used electrical energy to provide local heating of tissue.

It is important to understand how these various energy sources result in ablation of myocardial tissue. The mechanisms by which these various techniques create useful damage can be described as follows:

- the high energy techniques cause mechanical as well as electrical damage;

- the low energy techniques cause primarily electrical damage;

- RF ablation causes thermal damage;

- transcoronary ablation acts via chemical toxicity; and

- microwave radiation causes primarily thermal damage.

The predominant mechanisms by which cardiac cells are damaged using various ablation techniques are illustrated in Figure 1.

High energy application causes a rather large and irregular lesion,[11] which results from mechanical stress to the cells induced by a shock wave (barotrauma). Application of low energy direct current (D.C.) shocks causes a relatively large area of damage through electroporation of cell membranes, a process in which electrical current causes irreversible structural defects in the phospholipid layers that maintain the structural integrity of cells.[12]

Radiofrequency ablation damages cells primarily through heating, which occurs through conduction of heat away from the hottest area close to the electrode tip (conductive and convective heating), and also, to a lesser extent, by heat generated in the tissue by the RF currents (direct heating). The area of damage is typically small and clearly demarcated.

Principles of Catheter Ablation • 189

barotrauma	electroporation	direct and indirect heating
HIGH ENERGY	LOW ENERGY	RF

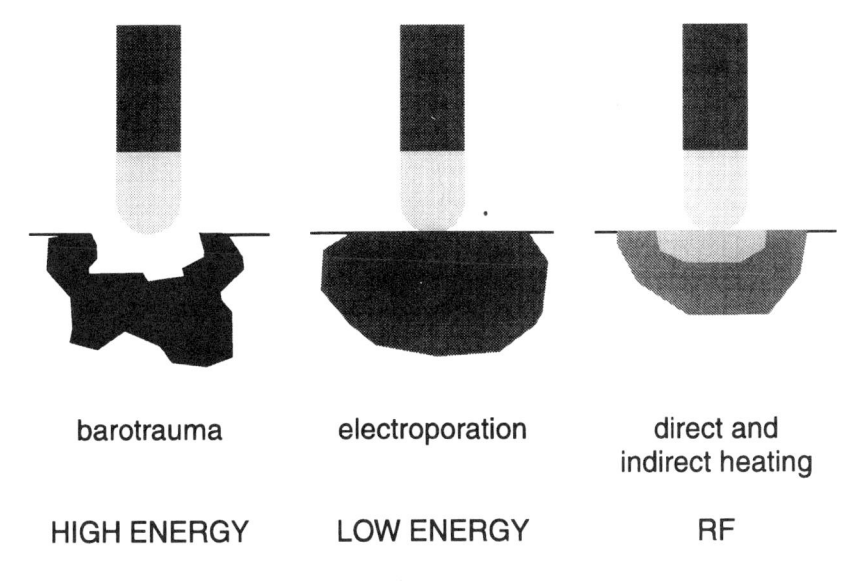

Figure 1. *The principal mechanisms of damage by high energy, low energy, and RF ablation.*

High Energy Ablation

The physical consequences of a high energy impulse are complex.[13-15] The electrode is initially insulated by gas formed by electrolysis. If the voltage on the electrode is still high, electrical arcing may take place. Six phases may then be identified (Fig. 2), as follows:

1. heating and electrolysis;
2. insulation and arcing;
3. rapid expansion of a vapor globe, in a fashion analogous to that of an explosion;
4. arc extinction and terminal expansion of the vapor globe, followed by
5. rapid collapse producing a shock wave with microbubble formation (cavitation); and
6. return to initial resistive current flow.

The lesion produced by this violent physical process is not only large, but the physical effects of the discharge may be widespread, extending throughout the heart. The diffuse nature of myocardial damage that results from these energies is the consequence of the cavitation effect that follows in the wake of the shock wave as it travels through the heart.

1. heating and electrolysis

2. insulation and arcing

3. rapid vapour globe expansion

4. arc extinction
terminal expansion

surface of vapour globe acts as "virtual electrode"

5. rapid collapse, shock wave production

microbubbles (cavitation)

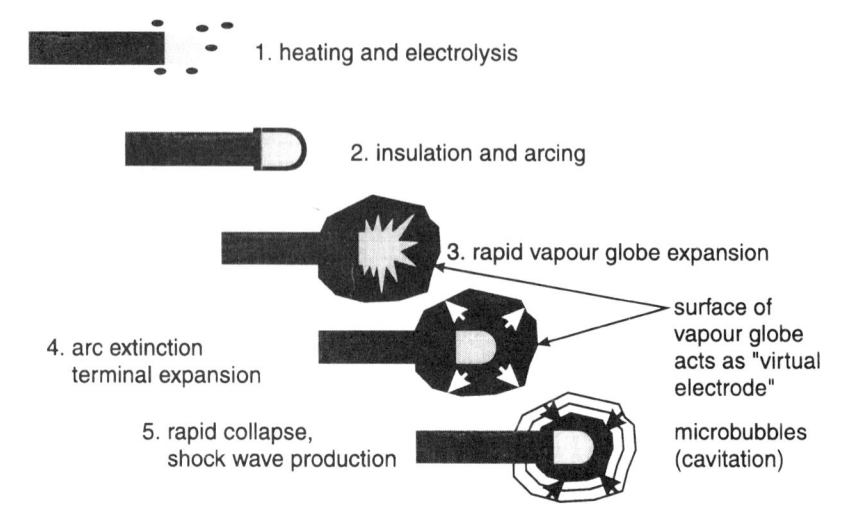

Figure 2. *The effects of a high energy impulse.*

Low Energy Ablation

While the extent of tissue damage caused by high energy impulses (D.C. shocks) is mainly determined by the expansion of the vapor globe, the size of the lesion caused by low energy catheter ablation depends on the electrical field strength, thus on current density, in the tissue.

Figure 3 illustrates how the electrical field falls off rapidly with increasing distance from the axis of the catheter, which is equipped with a 4 mm electrode in this example. The electrical field will cause holes in the cell membrane (electroporation), leading to cell death, when a certain level, indicated in Figure 3 by a horizontal line at 20%, is exceeded.

The passing of current through a resistive medium, such as myocardial tissue, causes transformation of electrical into thermal energy. Low energy ablation will therefore also cause local tissue heating. In Figure 4, the influence of the distance from the catheter axis on direct heating by the ablation current is illustrated. It is a relatively unimportant factor in the application of high and low energy ablation shocks because damage caused by barotrauma and electroporation typically extends much further from the electrode than that caused by tissue heating.

Principles of Catheter Ablation • 191

4mm electrode

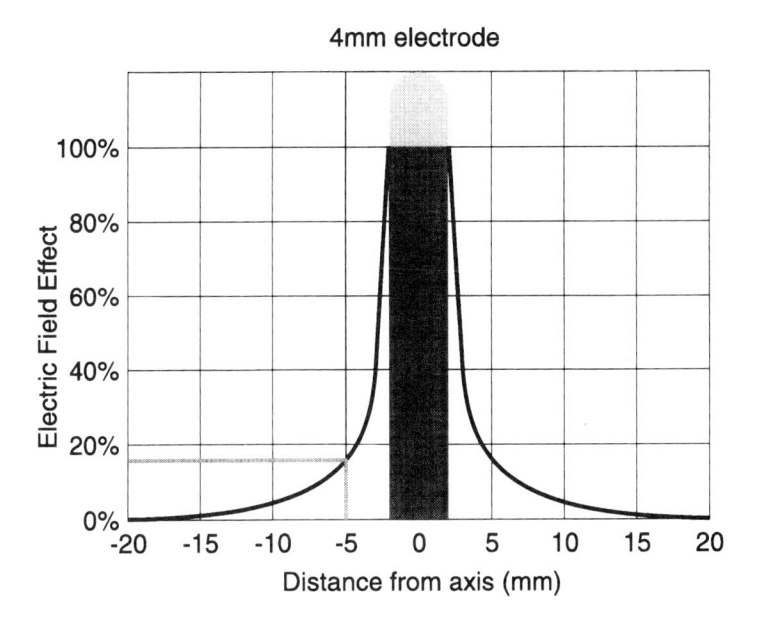

Figure 3. *Electrical field strength, responsible for electroporation when a certain level is exceeded, falls off rapidly as a function of distance from the electrode.*

FIELD EFFECT
Electric and Direct Thermal

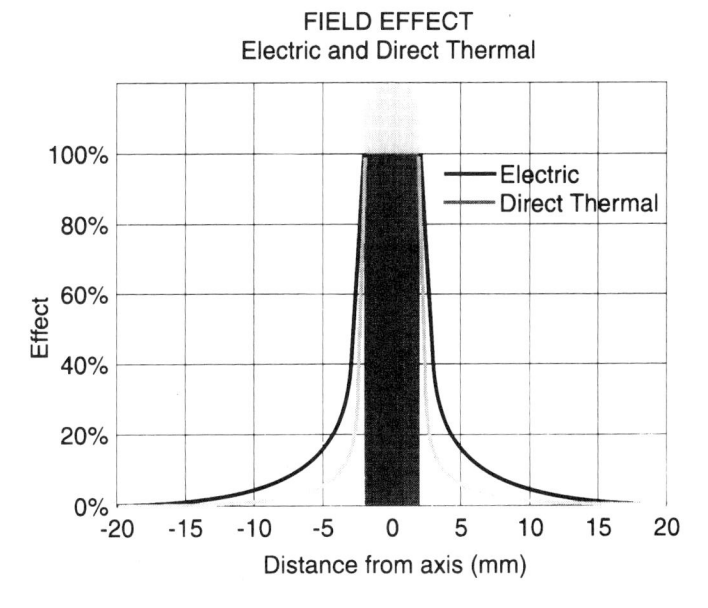

Figure 4. *The extent of tissue damage caused by electrical (electroporation) and by thermal effects during low energy ablation.*

Radiofrequency Ablation

Figure 5 depicts the temperature gradient developing around a RF catheter electrode of 4 mm diameter, heated to about 100°C at the interface between metal and tissue. While current passes through the tissues surrounding the electrode, local, direct heating occurs to a degree proportional to the local dissipation of electrical energy.

Because current density is highest in the immediate vicinity of the electrode, heating is at its maximum there, as it is for all forms of catheter ablation using electrical energy. The effect of this direct electrical heating of the tissues falls off rather sharply with distance from the electrode, and the area in which the temperature will rise to about 55°C, the level at which permanent cell damage will occur, does not extend much further away than about 1 mm from the electrode. This explains why an RF lesion is relatively small.

Heat is passively conducted from warmer to colder areas, with heat flow determined by temperature gradients and local heat conduction properties of the tissue. Figure 6 illustrates the effect of this secondary, passive heating during RF ablation due to heat conduction away from the electrode tip. This passive heating slightly increases the area of cell damage by about 30% in cross-section and by about 50% in total volume. The effect of damage caused by heat conduction depends importantly on the contact between the electrode and the tissue, and on the heat conduction properties of the tissue and blood surrounding the electrode. Poor contact between the electrode and tissue results in dissipation of heat into the blood pool, cooling of the electrode, and little rise in myocardial temperature. Loss of heat due to convection also affects the shape of the myocardial lesion. The surface layer adjacent to the electrode will be cooled by the passage of blood more than the deeper layers and, therefore, the lesion will be at its broadest at some distance into the tissue.

The size of the RF lesion is increased by passive heating, which may result in progressive electrode intrusion into the tissue when the contact pressure on the electrode is high. This leads to a further increase in the volume, especially depth, that may result in damage to valves, the coronary sinus, and other cardiac structures. The limitation on energy transfer using RF may occur because of coagulation of blood on the electrode surface that occurs when the tip temperature rises too far. The increase in impedance prevents current flow and power drops. Cooling the electrode tip—cold saline flushing offers one method—prevents coagulum formation and allows greater power delivery and larger lesion volume.

Principles of Catheter Ablation • 193

TEMPERATURE GRADIENT
Direct Electrical Heating

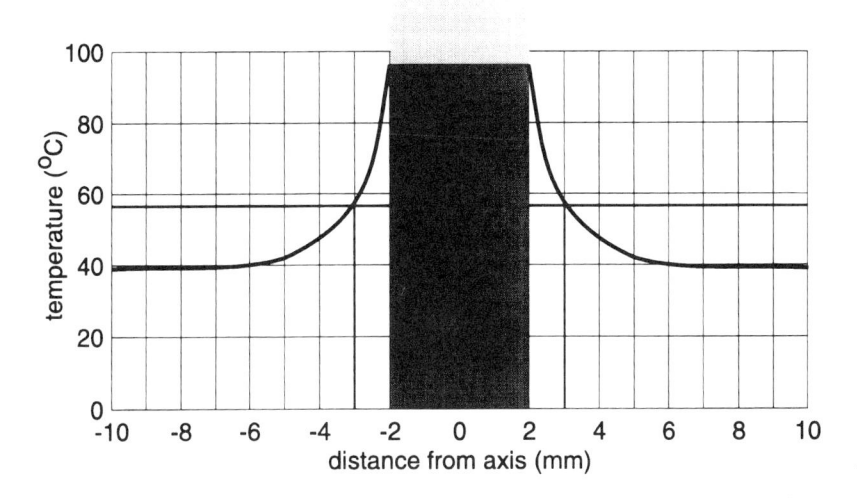

Figure 5. *Temperature gradient around an RF ablation electrode as caused by direct heating of the surrounding tissue due to current passage.*

TEMPERATURE GRADIENT
Direct and Passive Electrical Heating

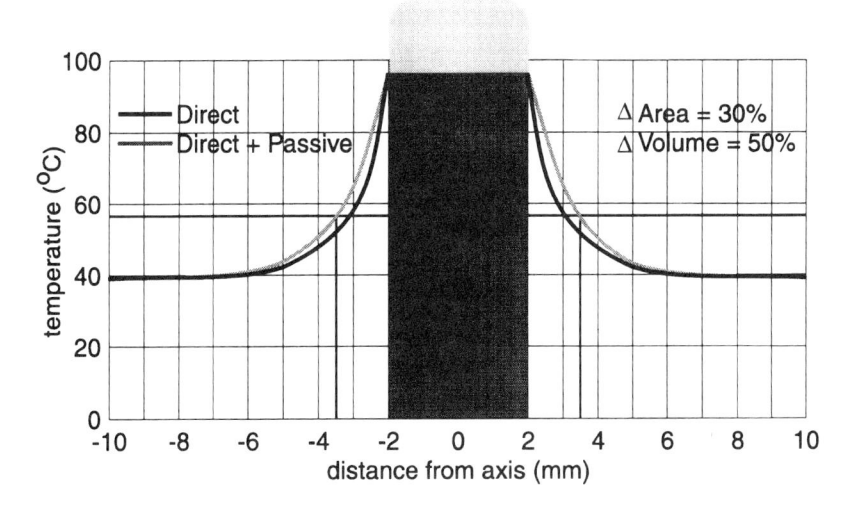

Figure 6. *Expansion of the tissue area raised above 55°C during RF ablation due to passive heat conduction.*

194 • TRANSVENOUS DEFIBRILLATION AND RF ABLATION

Figure 7 illustrates why the direct effect of the electrical field on cells (electroporation) extends further away from the electrode surface than the effects caused by local heating: the electrical field falls off with increasing distance from the electrode surface in proportion to the distance squared and the local heating caused by the local electrical field is proportional to the square of the electrical field strength, thus falling off with the fourth power of the distance. This explains why the lesion caused by RF ablation, primarily due to heating effects in the tissue, is smaller than the lesion caused by high energy electrical shocks, which is primarily due to electrical effects.

The main mechanisms of inducing cell damage and their dependence on distance from the ablation electrode are summarized in Figure 8 for high energy, low energy, and RF ablation.

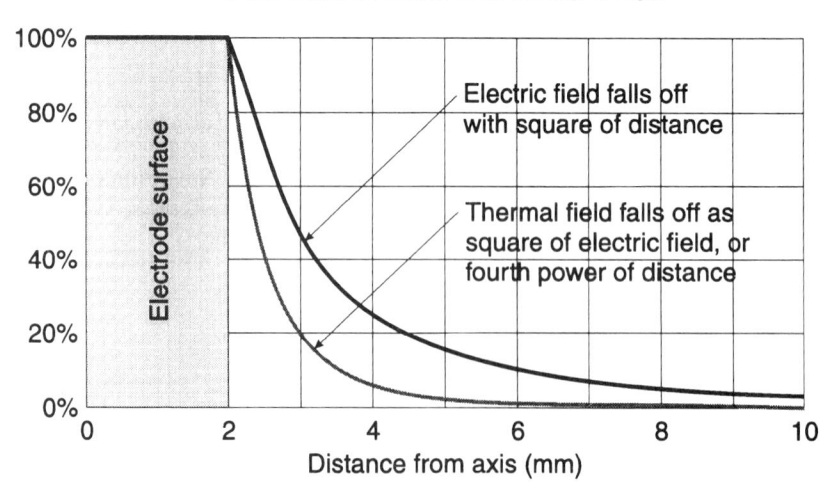

Figure 7. *Direct electrical and thermal effects of ablation currents as a function of distance from the electrode.*

Principles of Catheter Ablation • 195

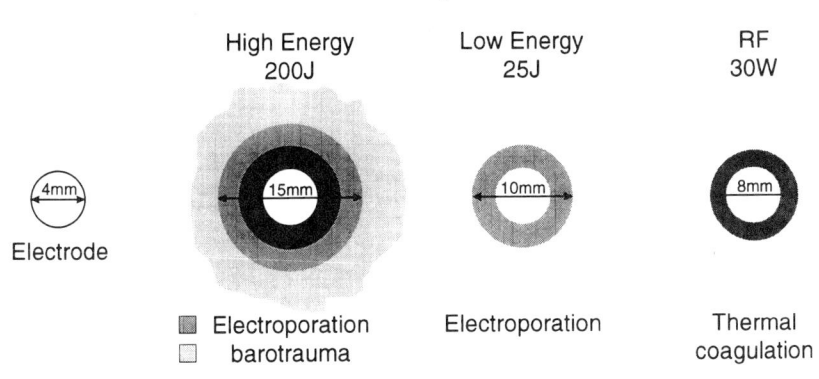

Figure 8. *Mechanisms and extent of cell damage during high energy, low energy, and RF ablation.*

Advantages and Disadvantages of Various Energy Sources

High energy ablation has the advantage that the energy source, an external defibrillator, is readily available. Its main disadvantages are that the results are unpredictable, that its safety record is questionable, and that general anesthesia is required.

The advantages of low energy ablation are that it causes a relatively small enzyme rise, that the volume of its lesion is large compared to that induced by RF ablation, and that it has proven to be an efficacious technique. The disadvantages are that general anesthesia is required and that a special energy source needs to be available.

The advantages of RF ablation are that general anesthesia is not required and that it has proven to be highly effective in various applications. The disadvantages are that the lesion volume is small and that the electrode therefore has to be very close to the target lesion.

Transcoronary ablation has as an advantage that general anesthesia is not necessary and that, in the case of ablation of the AV node, electrophysiological mapping of the AV junction is not strictly required. Its disadvantages are that it produces an unpredictable lesion, that selective cannulation of coronary vessels is required, and that its safety record has not yet been established.

Ablation with microwave energy is still in an experimental stage. It has the potential advantages that it may not require general anesthesia, that the lesion volume may be large, and that the energy can be applied in a directional fashion. Potential disadvantages or possible uncertainties are that catheters for microwave ablation have not yet been proven safe and that failure modes are presently uncertain.

At present, RF ablation is the most acceptable method for the patient, provides the most controllable method of creating localized myocardial damage, and should be used whenever its success rate is adequate. Accessory AV pathway ablation and slow pathway ablation should always use RF energy as the initial energy with low energy as a backup for accessory AV pathway ablation. Experience with RF energy for ablation of AV conduction is more limited but there is increasing evidence that it is the technique of first choice with low energy D.C. current providing an effective alternative.

High energy ablation of ventricular tachycardia (VT) carries a significant risk of complications. Other systems such as low energy ablation, alcohol ablation, and RF ablation have relatively low success rates or are yet to be validated, as is the case for microwave ablation.

The solutions to ablation of myocardial tissue for VT and atrial flutter will depend as much on improving techniques of mapping to define the critical zone of the arrhythmia as on developing new power sources and catheters.

Conclusions

The requirements for catheter ablation will depend on the type of arrhythmia and the underlying substrate. Radiofrequency energy is highly successful for ablation of accessory AV pathways. However, the question should be asked if it produces the correct type of lesion and if the nature of the lesion is not responsible for some of the complications such as endocarditis and thromboembolism. Other important questions are how radiation exposure can be reduced and if all centers can reproduce the success rates achieved by the presently experienced centers.

References

1. Gonzales R, Scheinman M, Margaretten W, et al: Closed chest electrode-catheter technique for His bundle ablation in dogs. Am J Physiol (Heart Circ Physiol) 1981; 241:H283-H288.
2. Scheinman MM, Morady F, Hess DS, et al: Catheter-induced ablation of the atrioventricular junction to control refractory supraventricular arrhythmias. JAMA 1982; 248:851-855.

3. Cunningham AD, Rowland E, Rickards AF: A new low energy power source for catheter ablation. PACE 1986; 9:1384-1388.
4. Borggrefe M, Budde T, Podczeck A: High frequency alternating current ablation of an accessory pathway in humans. J Am Coll Cardiol 1987; 10:576-582.
5. Langberg JJ, Chin MC, Lee MA, et al: Ablation of the atrioventricular junction with radiofrequency energy: Improved results with a new electrode catheter. J Am Coll Cardiol 1990; 15:133A. Abstract.
6. Brugada P, de Swart H, Smeets J, et al: Transcoronary chemical ablation of ventricular tachycardia. Circulation 1989; 79:475-482.
7. Sneddon JF, Linker NJ, O'Nunain S, et al: Transcoronary atrioventricular nodal modification using microvascular collagen. PACE 1991; 14:1976-1980.
8. Salerno J, Narula OS, Finzi A, et al: Electro-thermal modulation of A-V conduction in junctional tachycardias: Short-term and long-term results. Eur Heart J 1990; 6:163. Abstract.
9. Hidden F, Lavergne T, Verdier J, et al: Transvenous modification of canine atrioventricular conduction using a cryogenic catheter. Eur Heart J 1990; 11:62. Abstract.
10. Langberg JJ, Wonnell T, Chin MC, et al: Catheter ablation of the atrioventricular junction using a helical microwave antenna: A novel means of coupling energy to the endocardium. PACE 1991; 14:2105-2113.
11. Hauer RN, Straks W, Borst C, et al: Electrical catheter ablation in the right and left ventricular wall in dogs: Relation between delivered energy and histopathologic changes. J Am Coll Cardiol 1986; 8:637-643.
12. Jones JL, Lepeschkin E, Jones RE, et al: Response of cultured myocardial cells to countershock-type electric field stimulation. Am J Physiol 1978; 235:H214-H222.
13. Boyd EGCA, Holt PM: An investigation into the electrical ablation technique and a method of electrode assessment. PACE 1985; 8:815-823.
14. Bardy GH, Coltorti F, Ivey TD, et al: Some factors affecting bubble formation with catheter-mediated defibrillator impulses. Circulation 1986; 73:525-538.
15. Cunningham AD, Rowland E, Ahsan AJ, et al: Mechanism and significance of shock wave and gas production during catheter ablation. New Trends Arrhythmias 1988; 4:885-892.

21

Treatment of "Mahaim" Tachycardias by Radiofrequency Catheter Ablation

D.W. Davies

Historical Background

Accessory nodoventricular connections were first described by Mahaim[1-3] before intracardiac study of clinical cardiac electrophysiology was possible. When such techniques became available, tachycardias with characteristics compatible with mediation by nodoventricular fibers were identified[4] (Table 1) and were accordingly labeled "Mahaim tachycardias." A clinicopathological correlation was provided later by antemortem electrophysiological study and subsequent postmortem histologic examination of an 11-year-old boy with recurrent paroxysmal left bundle branch block morphology tachycardias who did not recover consciousness after sinus rhythm was restored from ventricular fibrillation.[5]

Debate then developed as to the precise role of "Mahaim" fibers in the mediation of the tachycardias. The options were that the fibers formed the anterograde limb of a macroreentrant tachycardia[4] (Fig. 1A) or that they were merely a bystander to another (usually atrioventricular [AV] nodal) reentry circuit (Fig. 1B).[6]

From *Transvenous Defibrillation and Radiofrequency Ablation* edited by A. John Camm and Fred W. Lindemans © 1995, Futura Publishing Co., Inc., Armonk, NY.

Table 1
Essential Electrophysiological Characteristics of Mahaim Tachycardias

LBBB QRS morphology during tachycardia
Decremental anterograde A-H conduction
Decremental anterograde AV conduction
Shortening/reversal of H-V interval with increasing atrial prematurity
Negative H-V interval during tachycardia

Abbreviations: A-H: atrio-His; AV: atrioventricular; H-V: His-ventricular; LBBB: left bundle branch block.

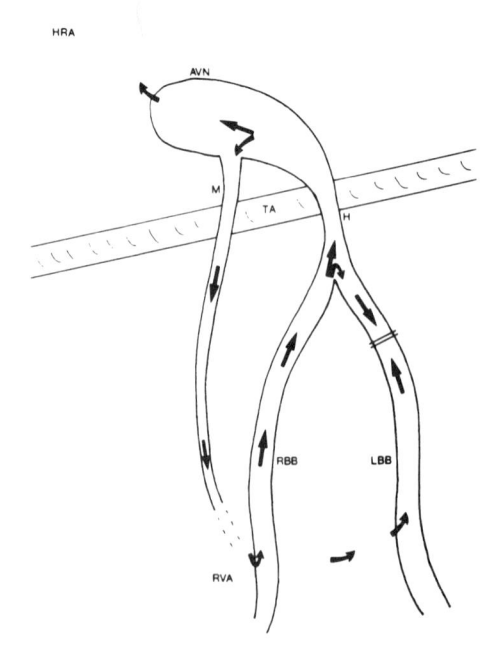

Figure 1A. *Diagram of a macroreentrant tachycardia involving a nodoventricular fiber as originally described by Mahaim. The "Mahaim" fiber conducts anterogradely, with activation returning retrogradely via the right bundle branch with collision and block in the left bundle branch. Abbreviations: AVN: atrioventricular node; H: His bundle; HRA: high right atrium; LBB: left bundle branch; M: "Mahaim" fiber; RBB: right bundle branch; RVA: right ventricular apex; TA: tricuspid annulus.*

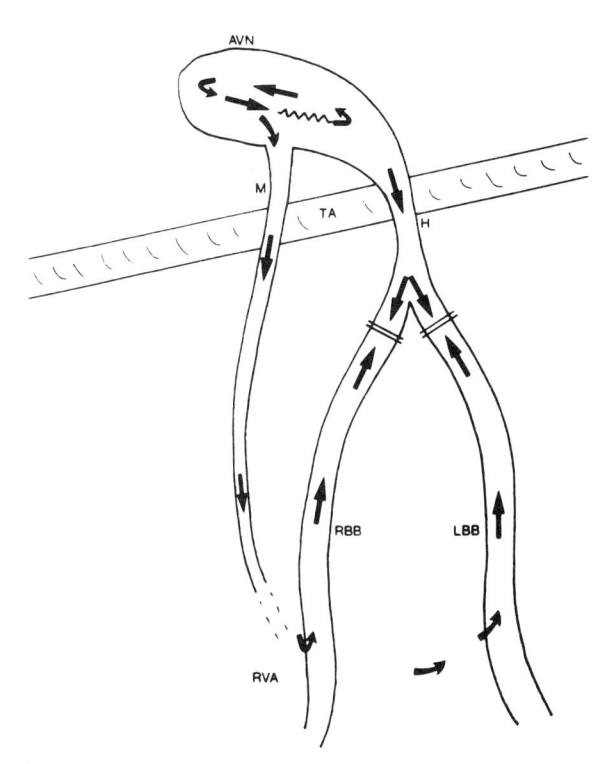

Figure 1B. *Diagram of AVNRT with bystander preexcitation by a nodoventricular fiber as originally described by Mahaim. Abbreviations: as for Figure 1A.*

Treatment of "Mahaim" Tachycardias

Despite the increased application of surgery to destroy accessory AV pathways, nodoventricular fibers were not treated in this way, presumably because it was thought that their intimate relationship to the AV node might have resulted in that structure also being damaged or destroyed. These tachycardias were therefore treated either by antiarrhythmic drugs (usually Class I)[4,7] or antitachycardia pacemakers.[5] Perhaps because of successful experience with curative surgery of AV nodal reentry tachycardia (AVNRT), a surgical approach to treating nine patients with "Mahaim" tachycardias was attempted.[8] In all cases, rather than nodoventricular fibers, the authors found decremental right parietal accessory pathways (Fig. 2) producing maximal right ventricular preexcitation at the "mid anterior" right ventricle in five of the nine patients. In the remaining four patients, the point of maximal right ventricular preexcitation was at the tricuspid annulus, compatible with a decremental right-sided "Kent" accessory pathway. In addition, five of the nine patients had additional AVNRT and two of the nine had an additional accessory AV pathway. The right free wall location of these decremental pathways and their frequent association with other junctional reentry circuits have been confirmed by numerous investigators[9,10] with the location of the "Mahaim" pathways being within the shaded area in Figure 3.

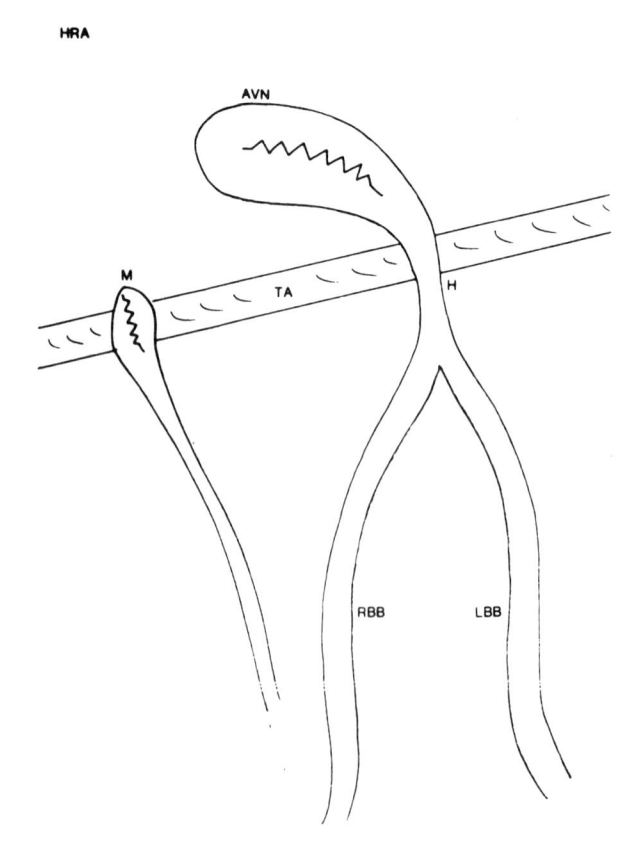

Figure 2. *Diagram of the "new" understanding of the connections associated with "Mahaim" electrophysiology showing a right free wall decremental accessory pathway (M). Abbreviations: AVN: atrioventricular node; H: His bundle; HRA: high right atrium; LBB: left bundle branch; M: "Mahaim" fiber; RBB: right bundle branch; TA: tricuspid annulus.*

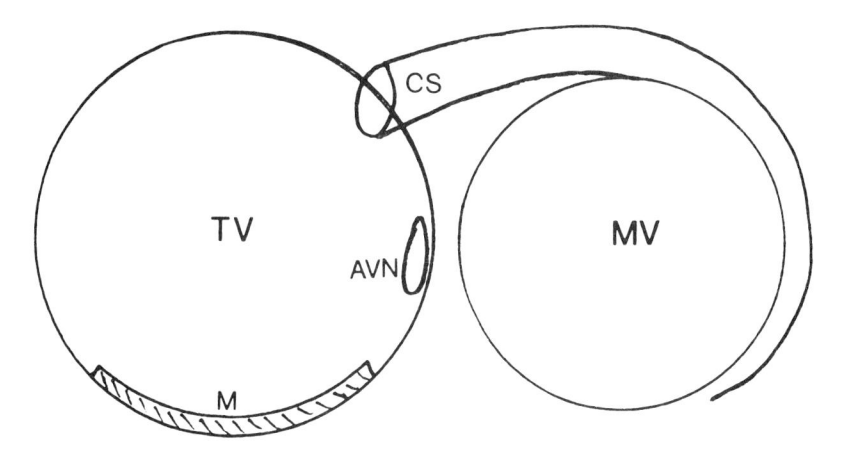

Figure 3. *Diagram showing the shaded area where "Mahaim" fibers are usually found on the anterior right free wall. Abbreviations: AVN: atrioventricular node; CS: coronary sinus; M: area for "Mahaim" fiber location; MV: mitral valve; TV: tricuspid valve.*

Catheter Ablation of "Mahaim" Tachycardias

Catheter delivered radiofrequency (RF) energy enables highly localized destruction of target tissue while preserving adjacent structures; e.g., the ablation of anteroseptal accessory pathways while conserving the adjacent AV node. With the development of increasingly steerable catheters, investigators can thus selectively destroy only the unwanted "accessory" pathways responsible for mediating junctional reentry tachycardias. The discovery that the accessory pathway in patients with "Mahaim" tachycardias is usually located at the tricuspid annulus on the right free wall has made these pathways easier targets for ablation techniques than they might have been as true "nodoventricular" pathways. However, particularly with the high incidence of other junctional reentry circuits found in these patients (Table 2),[8,9] it is important to ensure before targeting the pathway for ablation that it forms the anterograde limb of an antidromic AV reentry tachycardia (AVRT) rather than acting as a bystander to an alternative circuit. If the circuit is indeed a macroreentrant AVRT, then the retrograde limb to the AV node is likely to involve the right bundle branch (Fig. 4A). If conduction along this bundle was impaired by local trauma (catheter manipulation) and this led to either prolongation of tachycardia cycle length (by rerouting via the left bundle branch [Fig. 4B]) or its termina-

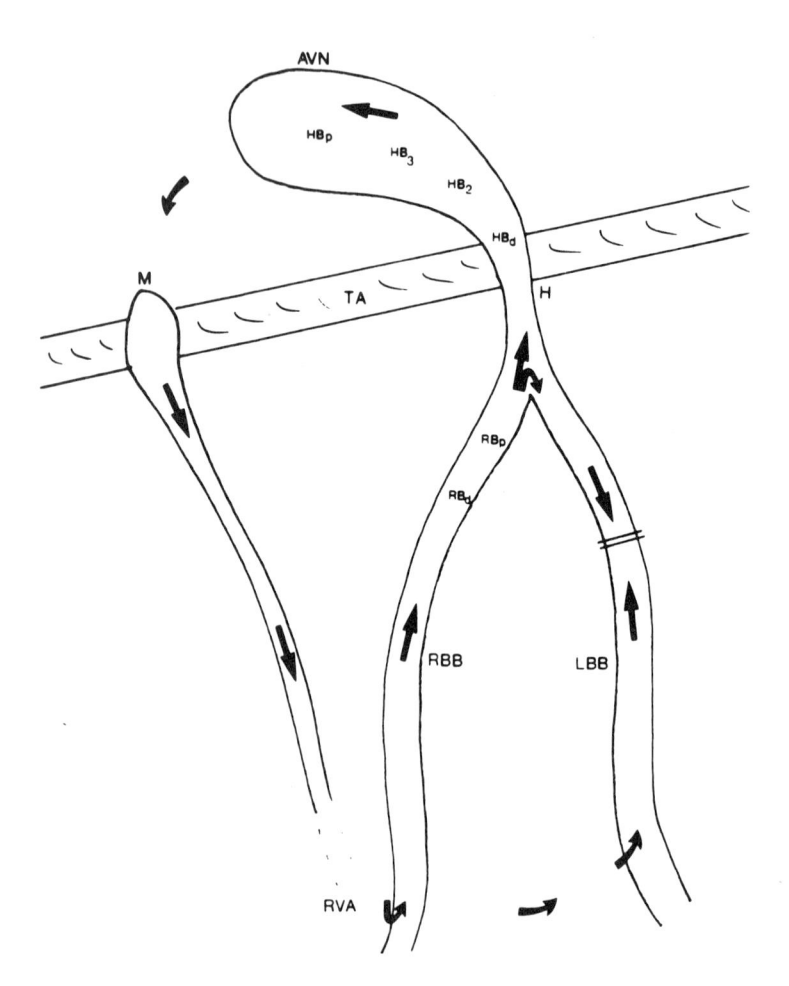

Figure 4A. *Diagram of macroreentrant circuit involving the decremental right free wall pathway as the anterograde limb, the right bundle branch as retrograde limb with collision, and block in the left bundle. Abbreviations: d: distal; HB: His bundle electrograms; p: proximal; AVN: atrioventricular node; H: His bundle; HRA: high right atrium; LBB: left bundle branch; M: "Mahaim" fiber; RB: right bundle; RBB: right bundle branch; RVA: right ventricular apex; TA: tricuspid annulus.*

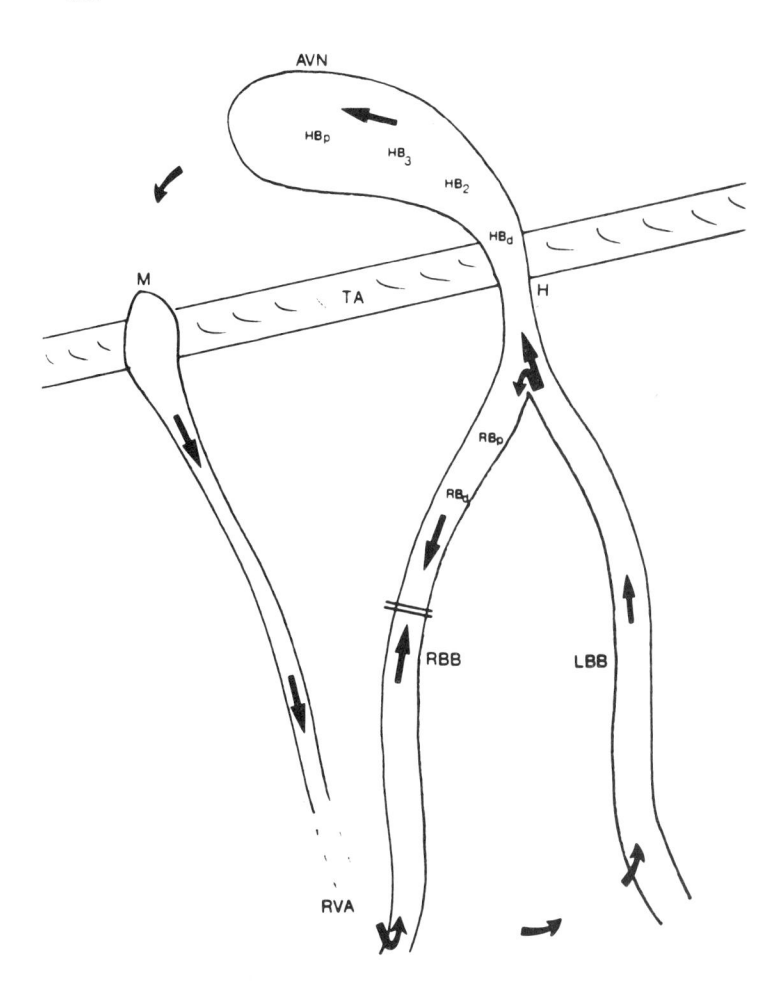

Figure 4B. *As for Figure 4A, but catheter manipulation had produced right bundle branch block so that, with a longer tachycardia cycle length, return is via the left bundle branch and the sequence of right bundle branch block is reversed. This disproves bystander preexcitation of AVNRT but would not affect the circuit if another accessory pathway was responsible for retrograde conduction to the atria. Abbreviations: d: distal; HB: His bundle electrograms; p: proximal; AVN: atrioventricular node; H: His bundle; HRA: high right atrium; LBB: left bundle branch; M: "Mahaim" fiber; RB: right bundle; RBB: right bundle branch; RVA: right ventricular apex; TA: tricuspid annulus.*

Table 2
Details of Radiofrequency Ablation for Seven Patients with "Mahaim" Pathways Successfully Ablated at St. Mary's, St. George's, and Royal Brompton and National Heart Hospitals, London, United Kingdom

Patient No.	Other JRT?	Other Cardiac Condition	Ablation Site
1	—	Ebstein's	TA
2	—	—	TA
3	PS AP	—	Sub TA
4	RFW AP	—	TA
5	—	—	TA
6	AVNRT	—	Sub TA
7	AVNRT	—	Fast pathway

Abbreviations: JRT: junctional reentry tachycardia; AVNRT: atrioventricular nodal reentry tachycardia; PS AP: posteroseptal accessory pathway; RFW AP: right free wall accessory pathway; TA: tricuspid annulus. For patient 7, "Mahaim" pathway activity was intermittent and its participation in tachycardia could not be proved. The common retrograde pathway for both tachycardias was therefore ablated with a good clinical result. However, this approach is not recommended because of the possibility of heart block and because of the possibility of retrograde slow AV nodal conduction leading to incessant tachycardia.

tion, then a macroreentrant mechanism, rather than bystander preexcitation of AVNRT, is proved.[4] Where the other potential circuit also involves an accessory pathway, then proof (by atrial activation mapping techniques) of the participation of that pathway in the junctional reentry circuit is sufficient to justify its ablation and this should be performed first if possible. The role of the "Mahaim" pathway in a possible reentry with the AV node as retrograde limb can then be assessed more clearly and the decision as whether or not to ablate the pathway can be made at that time.

For the pathways that simply bridge the tricuspid annulus, ablation has to be performed at that site. Electrograms obtained from these pathways are indistinguishable from classical AV nodal signals, consisting of an atrial deflection, followed after a delay (representing the pathway's decremental AV nodal-like properties) by a pathway deflection (similar to a His spike) and then by the ventricular deflection. Energy delivery at such sites on the tricuspid annulus will successfully destroy the pathway and usually be accompanied by a junctional rhythm, a hallmark of RF ablation of decremental tissue. This junctional rhythm can lead to instability of the catheter position particularly on the tricuspid annulus where catheter stability is notoriously difficult to achieve. Thus, for the longer pathways that appear to insert near the apical part of the right bundle branch, alternative sites of energy delivery may be considered.

On the pathway below the tricuspid annulus, the atrial component of the above signal is lost but the ventricular electrograms are preceded by a discrete spike when the ventricle is preexcited by the pathway. Energy delivery at the point of "insertion" of the pathway to the right bundle branch is always accompanied by permanent right bundle branch block.[9] This may not matter if the "Mahaim" pathway is also destroyed. However, if the right bundle branch alone is destroyed, then the longer tachycardia cycle length associated with return via the left bundle branch (Figs. 4A and 4B) allows a greater time for recovery of the node and of the pathway. On one occasion, this led to an incessant tachycardia requiring separate ablation of the "Mahaim" pathway at the tricuspid annulus in order to stop it (W. Jackman, personal communication). Thus, ablation at this site is not recommended. However, more proximal but subannular ablation sites have proved successful without any apparent disadvantage. Such sites, as with the apical sites, display ventricular electrograms preceded by a discrete spike that is seen only during ventricular preexcitation by the pathway, but is less likely to represent right bundle branch activity. Ectopic "junctional" rhythm is either minimal or not seen during energy delivery at such sites so that catheter stability is preserved. As with slow pathway ablation for cure of AVNRT, prolonged energy delivery may be required to destroy these pathways, irrespective of the site chosen for energy delivery.

Conclusions

The accessory pathways responsible for mediation of "Mahaim" tachycardias are not nodoventricular pathways but are decremental right free wall accessory pathways that usually appear to insert into the right bundle branch and are therefore best termed "atriofascicular" pathways. Although other junctional reentry circuits are often found in association, the pathway usually functions as the anterograde limb of an antidromic AVRT. It is therefore a suitable target for RF catheter ablation that is best achieved either at or under the tricuspid annulus. If an additional accessory pathway or an AVNRT circuit is present, then ablation of these is usually also necessary.

References

1. Mahaim I, Benatt A: Nouvelles recherches sur les connexions superieures de la branche gauche du faisceau de His-Tawara avec cloison interventriculaire. Cardiologia 1938; 1:61.
2. Mahaim I, Winston MR: Recherches d'anatomie comparee et de pathologie experimentale sur les connexions hautes du faisceau de His-Tawara. Cardiologia 1941; 5:189.
3. Mahaim I: Kent's fibers and the A-V paraspecific conduction through the upper connections of the bundle of His-Tawara. Am Heart J 1947; 33:651.
4. Gallagher JJ, Smith WM, Kasell JH, et al: Role of Mahaim fibers in cardiac arrhythmias in man. Circulation 1981; 64:176.
5. Gmeiner R, Ng CK, Hammer I, et al: Tachycardia caused by an accessory nodoventricular tract: A clinico-pathologic correlation. Eur Heart J 1984; 5:233.
6. Ward DE, Camm AJ, Spurrell RAJ: Ventricular preexcitation due to anomalous nodoventricular pathways: Report of 3 patients. Eur J Cardiol 1979; 9:111.
7. Lau CP, Davies DW, Mehta D, et al: Flecainide acetate in the treatment of tachycardias associated with Mahaim fibres. Eur Heart J 1987; 8:832.
8. Murdock C, Klein GJ, Guiraudon GM, et al: Epicardial mapping in patients with nodo-ventricular electrophysiologic pattern. Circulation 1990; 82(III):472.
9. Gursoy S, Schluter M, Duckeck W, et al: Radiofrequency current ablation in patients with Mahaim fibers. Eur Heart J 1992; 13(abs suppl):3.
10. Prior M, Beckman K, Moulton K, et al: Radiofrequency catheter ablation of Mahaim fibers at the tricuspid annulus. J Am Coll Cardiol 1991; 17:108A.

22

Radiofrequency Ablation of the Slow Pathway in Atrioventricular Nodal Reentrant Tachycardia: Electrogram Patterns at the Successful Site

B. Fischer, M. Haissaguerre, H. Pürerfellner, J.F. Warrin

Reentry in the atrioventricular (AV) node is the most common cause of regular paroxysmal supraventricular tachycardia. Radiofrequency (RF) catheter ablation of the slow pathway has been performed in patients with drug-refractory tachycardias. We have reported on the existence of peculiar slow potentials recorded from the midseptal and posteroseptal region in most humans. The prevalence of different electrogram patterns and their relation to a successful outcome are analyzed below.

Methods

One hundred fifty-one patients with the usual form of AV nodal reentrant tachycardia (AVNRT) were studied. Slow potentials were

From *Transvenous Defibrillation and Radiofrequency Ablation* edited by A. John Camm and Fred W. Lindemans © 1995, Futura Publishing Co., Inc., Armonk, NY.

defined as low amplitude activity (0.05 to 0.5 mV) prolonging or following atrial electrograms, needing high gain amplification (≥50 mm/mV) to become evident. They were recorded along a vertical band at the middle or posterior part of the septum near the tricuspid annulus. They occupied all or some of the diastolic interval between atrial electrogram and ventricular electrogram. Mostly, they were present during sinus rhythm, but sometimes they appeared only during atrial stimulation. However, their most specific pattern was their progressive response to increasing atrial rates that resulted in:

1. a separation from preceding atrial electrograms;
2. a dramatic decline in amplitude and slope; and
3. a corresponding increase in duration until, frequently, consistent activity disappears.

We have previously shown that such potentials do not represent atrial or Hissian activity.

Using a RF generator HAT™ 100 or 200 (Osypka, Germany), energy was applied during 90 seconds at a power of 40 W. Radiofrequency energy was delivered during sinus rhythm or atrial pacing. Ablation was performed at the site that showed both the most prominent slow potential (see below) and the absence of a significant (<0.1 mV) His bundle potential. If sustained AVNRT remained inducible, new RF applications were performed at contiguous sites. When a junctional rhythm occurred during RF delivery, AV conduction was assessed either by intermittent cessation of RF energy or by atrial overdrive pacing, particularly in midseptal sites.

Results

Electrograms at successful ablation sites are analyzed in Table I and illustrated in Figure 1. Overall clinical results of AVNRT ablation

Table 1
Various Electrogram Characteristics at Successful Ablation Sites

Multiple or fractionated atrial potentials <u>and</u> slow potentials	59%
Slow potentials	23%
Multiple or fractionated atrial potentials	15%
No complex potential	3%
Limitations: * contiguity of recording sites	
* catheter instability	
* interpretation of signal changes during pacing	

ELECTROGRAMS AT SUCCESSFUL ABLATION SITE

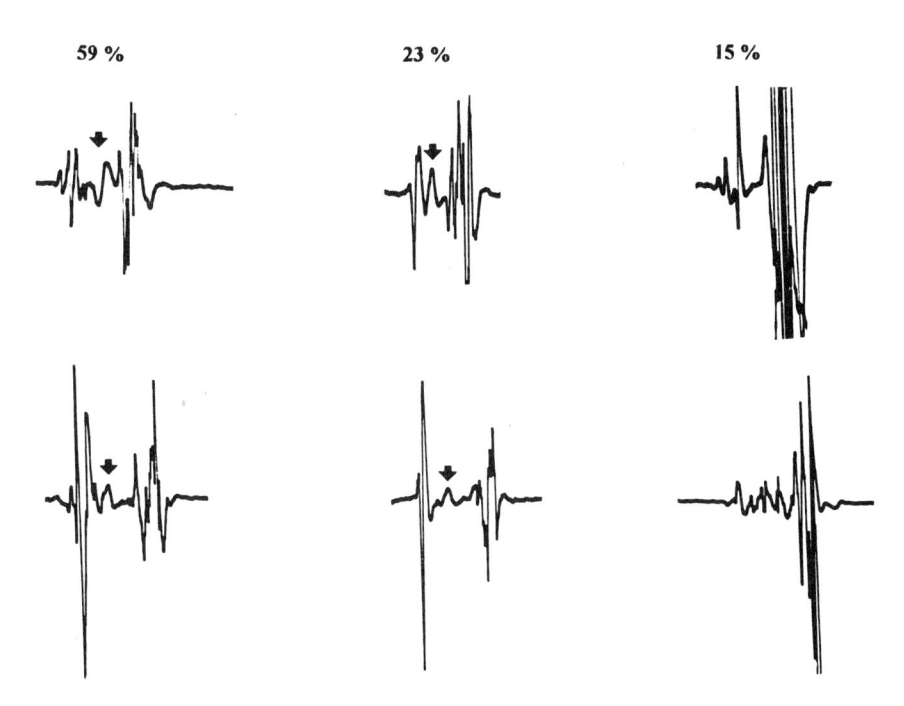

Figure 1. *Electrogram illustrations of multiple or fractionated atrial potentials* **and** *slow potentials as observed in 59% of successful ablation sites (left), slow potentials as observed in 23% of successful sites (middle), and multiple or fractionated atrial potentials observed in 15% of successful sites (right).*

Table 2
Results of Atrioventricular Nodal Reentrant Tachycardia
in 151 Patients

Ablation/Modification of Slow Pathway	Inadvertent or Deliberate Impairment of Fast Pathway
Median: 1–2 RF impulses N = 143 No AV block 3 clinical recurrences (2nd session) 1 failure	N = 8 1 AV block 2 clinical recurrences (2nd session)

in 151 patients are summarized in Table 2. In the last 70 patients, a median of one impulse was delivered. The time required for the catheter ablation procedure (the therapeutic component) was 41±38 minutes and fluoroscopy time was 14±14 minutes. No significant side effect was noted during the procedure. All patients preserved normal AV conduction except when there was inadvertent (n = 5) or deliberate (n = 3 patients with associated atrial arrhythmias) ablation of the fast pathway. One high degree AV block occurred during deliberate ablation of the fast pathway. Isolated echo beats remained inducible in 40% of patients. The main changes of the electrophysiological effects of ablation concerned the maximal value of the AH interval (340± 99 milliseconds versus 213±70 milliseconds). In 69% of the patients, post-ablation atrial stimulation could not achieve a long AH interval, which previously was critical for tachycardia induction or maintenance. All patients but one were free of tachycardias in the absence of treatment over a follow-up period of 1 to 28 months.

Discussion

This study analyzes different endocardial electrogram pattern characteristics and their relation to a successful clinical outcome. The most striking finding is the presence of both multiple or fractionated atrial electrograms and so-called slow potentials in 59% of successful ablation sites. Whereas their isolated occurrence is less predictive for a favorable ablation result, their combination leads to a significant rise in the success rate of ablation of AVNRT. It is very important to note that slow potentials must have two characteristics, as discussed below.

1. They need high gain amplification (50 to 100 mm/mV) to be recorded.
2. They may be confused with "ordinary" atrial electrograms (or even His bundle potentials) and therefore need to be further assessed by atrial pacing techniques (Figs. 2A through 2D illustrate these phenomena). With atrial pacing, they separate from preceding atrial electrograms and progressively alter. Catheter instability is the main limiting factor to reliably record and interpret circumscribed electrical activities and to study the various anatomical structures involved. In fact, the proximal atrionodal region ("the transitional node") is a heterogeneous mixture of atrial muscle and AV nodal fibers. It is probable that the simultaneous recording through the same electrode of

complex atrial and slow potentials clearly expresses this heterogeneity, probably representing the substrate for a prenodal slow conducting system. Slow versus spike potentials may express either anatomical (AV nodal versus atrial activity) or functional differences: transverse anisotropic versus longitudinal transmitted wavefronts.

Conclusion

By using discrete potentials in the proximal atrionodal region as a target for RF energy, almost complete clinical success in the ablation or modification of slow pathway conduction in patients presenting with AVNRT was achieved. No block occurred with this approach, in contrast to ablation of the fast pathway.

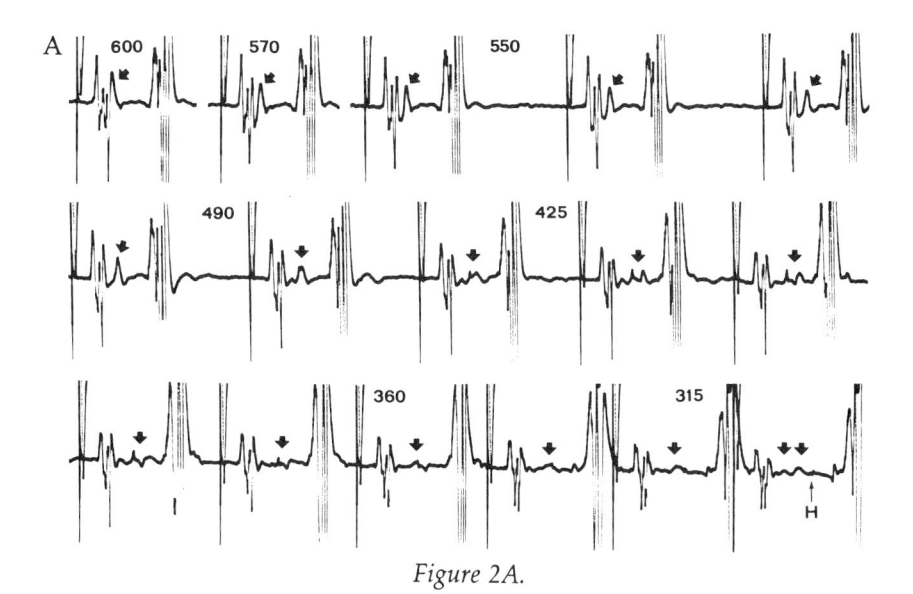

Figure 2A.

Figure 2B.

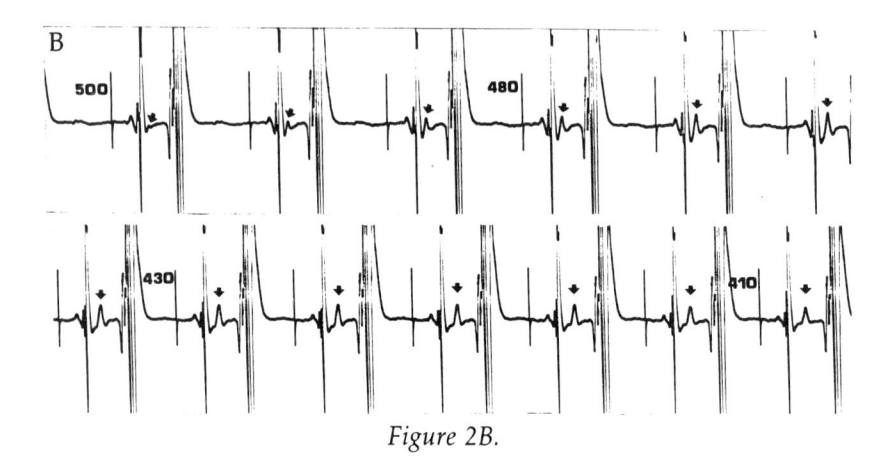

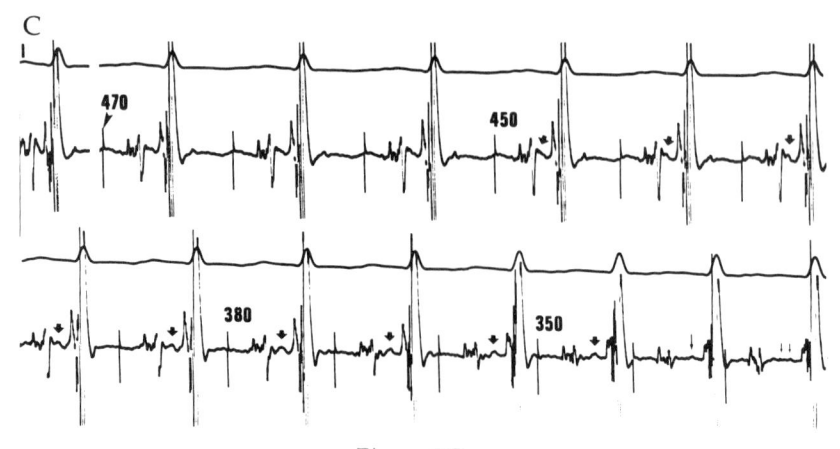

Figure 2C.

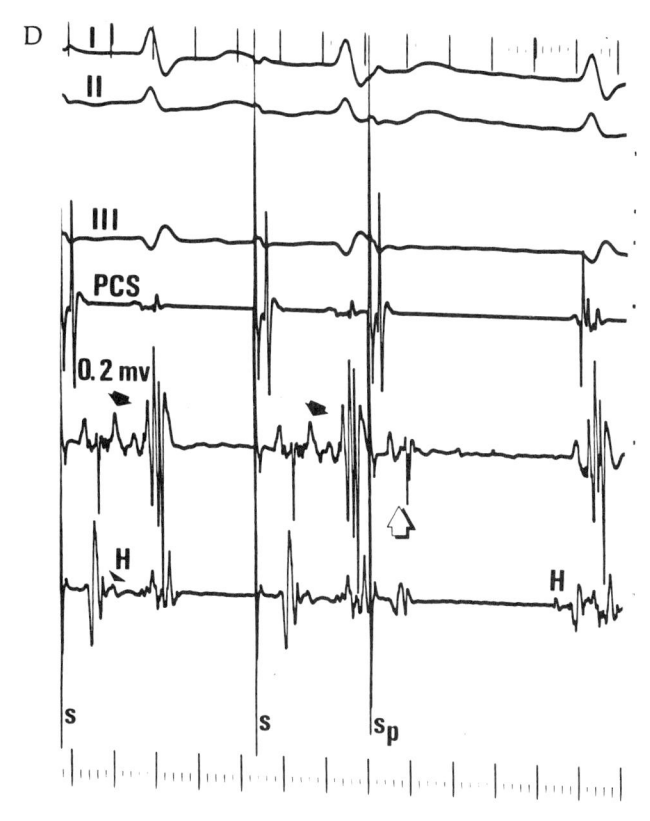

Figure 2A-D. *The effects of shortening atrial pacing intervals on the characteristic multiple/fractionated atrial electrograms and slow potentials, as observed in 59% of successful ablation sites.*

23

Radiation Exposure during Radiofrequency Ablation of Accessory Pathways

M. Fromer, J. Schläpfer

Percutaneous catheter ablation of accessory pathways using radiofrequency (RF) current has become a common method for curing patients with recurrent arrhythmias due to accessory pathway conduction. With this technique, between 80% and 100% of patients can be permanently cured of their congenital abnormality. Acute mortality and morbidity of the intervention are low. For these reasons, catheter ablation has become the therapy of choice for patients with symptomatic reentrant tachycardias due to an accessory pathway and it has almost completely replaced the surgical intervention.

Catheter ablation requires precise localization of the accessory pathways, which is accomplished using fluoroscopy guidance for placing the catheter at the right- or left-sided atrioventricular (AV) groove. As RF ablation creates only small circumscript lesions, the ultimate catheter position must be guided by recording of the intracardiac signals indicating accessory pathway conduction. Catheter placement can be difficult and time consuming, which is responsible for long fluoroscopy times. This represents radiation exposure for the patient as well as for the physician and is therefore a potential long-term risk for the development of malignancies or genetic defects. As patients undergo-

From *Transvenous Defibrillation and Radiofrequency Ablation* edited by A. John Camm and Fred W. Lindemans © 1995, Futura Publishing Co., Inc., Armonk, NY.

ing RF ablation for accessory pathways are usually young, it is of special interest to analyze the long-term safety of this method.

It is important to realize that radiation exposure may originate from the primary beam as well as from secondary, scattered radiation and that the risks are age and gender dependent.

Review of the Literature

From a review of the literature, it becomes quite clear that the first studies dealing with RF ablation had no concerns regarding exposure to x-rays during the procedure. More recent studies on RF ablation provide data concerning the amount of radioscopy exposure.

Schlüter et al,[1] Calkins et al,[2] and Lesh et al[3] reported on series of respectively 92, 250, and 100 patients in whom accessory pathways in various locations were ablated. The mean radioscopy times±SD were 54±33, 47±33, and 66±8 minutes, respectively.

A paper by Kuck and Schlüter[4] deals exclusively with left lateral accessory pathways in 34 patients, with the single catheter approach leading to a short radioscopy time: 23±20 minutes.

Lemery et al[5] used a modified direct current (D.C.) shock instead of RF current to ablate accessory pathways in 35 patients. Their study indicates that fluoroscopy time may vary according to the location of the accessory pathway: 46±24 minutes for the left free wall and 66±33 minutes for other locations. Chen et al[6] compared the efficacy of D.C. shock ablation to RF ablation. They started their learning experience with D.C. shock in this patient group. The average radioscopy time was 12 minutes shorter compared to ablations with RF current. According to another study by Schlüter and Kuck,[7] radioscopy time was 44±25 minutes in 12 patients with anteroseptal accessory pathways. Radioscopy time was unfortunately not indicated in several important papers. Figure 1 summarizes the radioscopy times for RF ablation as reported by these various authors.

Two groups of authors paid special attention to the radioscopy exposure during RF ablation. Lindsay et al[8] analyzed x-ray exposure in detail in 64 patients and Calkins et al[9] studied x-ray exposure in 31 patients.

In Lindsay's[8] group, about half of the patients underwent RF ablation for AV nodal reentry tachycardia. They found that the average effective dose-equivalent of 1.7 rem for a patient undergoing ablation is between the dose-equivalent during coronary angiography (1.2 rem) and percutaneous transluminal coronary angioplasty (2.2 rem) or thal-

Comparison of radioscopy times (min) for RF ablation

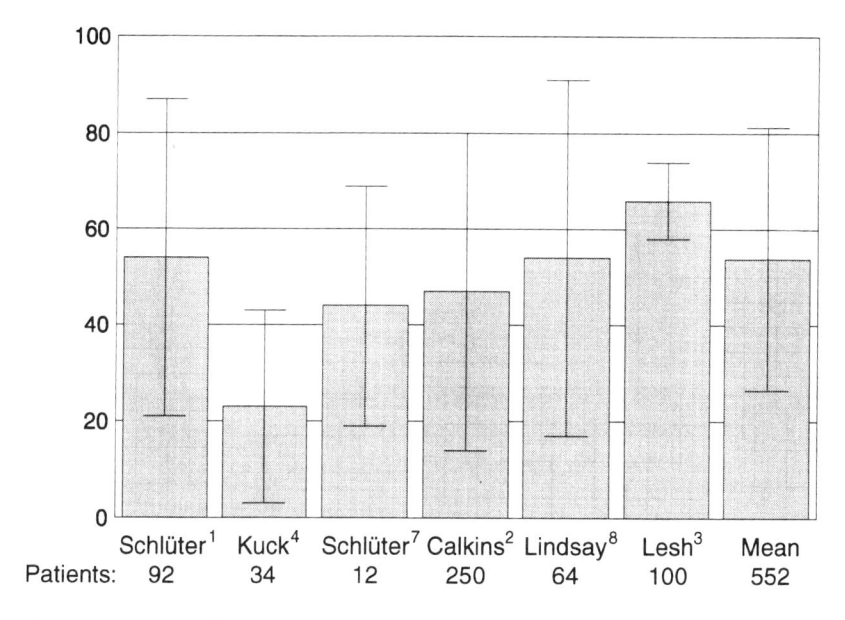

Figure 1. *Mean radioscopy times±1 SD for RF ablation as reported by various authors.*

lium scintigraphy (2.1 rem). The recommended annual maximum dose for personnel is listed as 5.0 rem. The average annual natural dose in the United States is 0.3 rem. The authors stated that about 55 minutes of fluoroscopy time may increase the risk of fatal cancer to 1 in 745 cases, which is an increase of 1% of the spontaneous risk.

In the study by Calkins et al,[9] the physicians involved in the investigation were all experienced in the technique of ablation. The primary beam was collimated and an additional shield between physician and image intensifier was available. The highest measured exposure rates in the patients were: 447 mrem/minute at the ninth vertebra, 64 mrem/minute at the posterior illiac crest, and 58 mrem/minute at the anterior xyphoid. The left hand (2.25 mrem/minute) is the physician's most exposed component. The ablator's waist received an average 1.21 mrem/minute outside the lead protection and no measurable dose underneath the lead. The physician's left maxilla received 0.53 mrem/minute, the thyroid was exposed to 0.36 mrem/minute outside, and to no measurable dose underneath the lead protection. In their conclusions, the authors estimated that conventional fluoroscopic imaging is associated with a lifetime risk of developing a fatal malignancy of 1 per 1000 patients per hour of fluoroscopy.

We also analyzed the radioscopy exposure at our institution. The results were comparable to those of Calkins et al.[9] The exposure measured to the patient's thyroid, however, was almost 10 times smaller than indicated by Calkins et al.[9] Almost the same was true for the exposure to the posterior iliac crest of the patient and the exposure to the left hand of the operator was also considerably smaller. The reason for these differences can be explained as follows: more effective shielding between primary source and scattered radiation; protection of the thyroid and of the gonad area of the patient (the exposure to the iliac crest is used to estimate gonad exposure); and lack of standardization of the measurement sites resulting in small differences in the placement of the x-ray sensitive dose collectors. As the exposure drops rapidly as a function of distance, small differences may have an important impact on the registered doses.

When we analyze the local experience concerning radioscopy exposure, it became quite obvious that radioscopy time is influenced by the localization of the accessory pathways. In 22 patients, the pathway was located at the left lateral free wall and the mean radioscopy time was 39 minutes for ablation. With the exception of two cases, radioscopy time was smaller than or equal to 60 minutes. However, in two cases, excessive radioscopy time occurred. See Figure 2 for the scatter diagram.

In 51 patients with accessory pathways in other than left lateral localizations, fluoroscopy times showed a substantial scatter with a mean value of 59 minutes. In 21 cases, radioscopy times exceeded 60 minutes, and in one case it exceeded 160 minutes (see Fig. 3).

Conclusions and Recommendations

From the review of the literature and from our own experience, we conclude that the fluoroscopy time is influenced by the localization of the target pathway, by the type of energy applied to ablate the pathway, by the effort made to use shielding for protecting the patient and the physician, by the catheter material, and by the experience of the operators.

X-ray exposure can be considerably reduced by applying gonad and thyroid protection of the patient, the use of radioprotective shields, the collimation of the radiographic beam, and the use of pulsed fluoroscopy.

Fluoroscopy time for ablation of left lateral AP

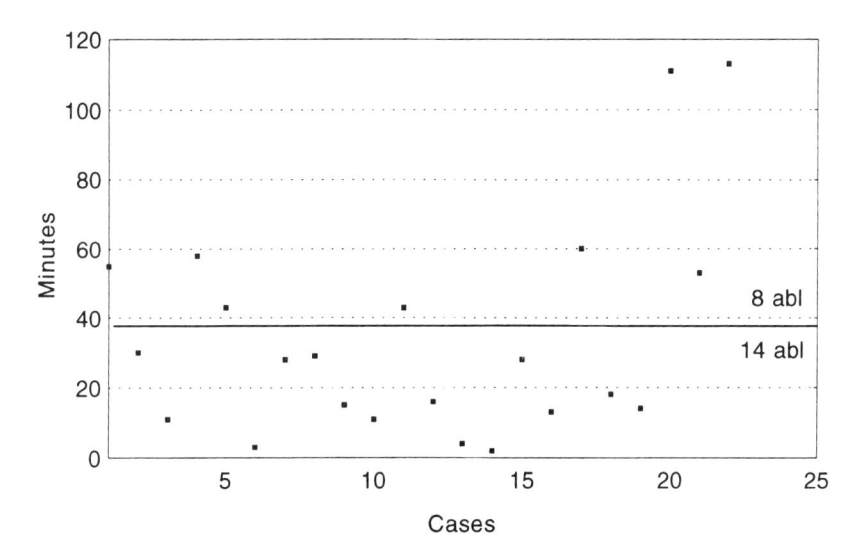

Figure 2. *Fluoroscopy times in 22 RF ablation procedures for left-lateral accessory pathways. AP: accessory pathway.*

It is strictly recommended to avoid angiography and to stop procedures after 60 minutes of fluoroscopy. There is no doubt that the actual state of the technique exposes the young patient to a small increase of the risk to experience a fatal malignancy during his or her lifetime. This risk is different for various organs. The most serious risk for female patients is the development of breast cancer. According to our measurements, this risk might be one to two cases per 1000 ablations exceeding 60 minutes of fluoroscopy.

Therefore, the best precautions are the following:

1. ablation should be performed only by experienced teams;
2. pulsed fluoroscopy, which reduces the exposure by about 40%, should be used instead of conventional fluoroscopy;
3. careful lead protection should be applied to reduce scattered beam radiation;
4. collimation of the primary beam should be used; and
5. the patient's thyroid and gonad areas should be protected with lead.

Fluoroscopy time for ablation of right sided AP and left, but not of left lateral AP

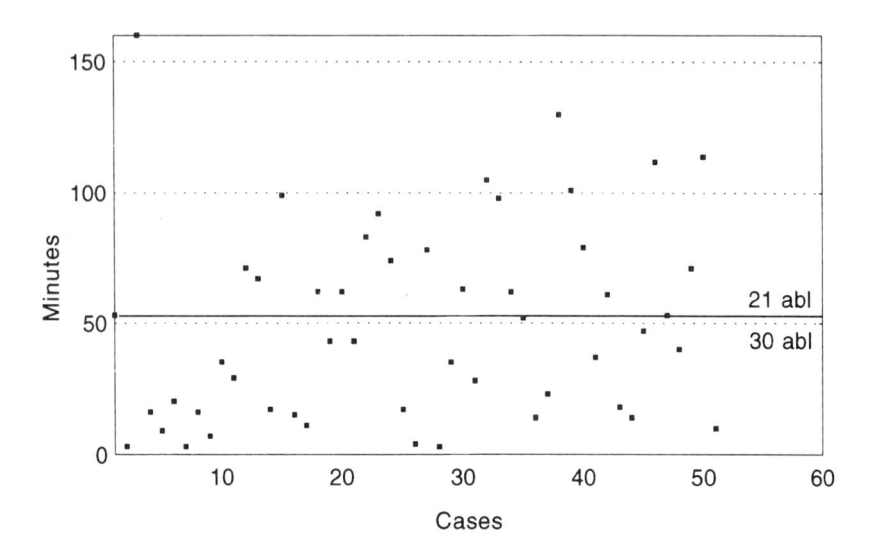

Figure 3. *Fluoroscopy times in 51 RF ablation procedures for right- and left-sided, excluding left-lateral, accessory pathways. AP: accessory pathway.*

References

1. Schlüter M, Geiger M, Siebels J, et al: Catheter ablation using radiofrequency current to cure symptomatic patients with tachyarrhyhtmias related to an accessory atrioventricular pathway. Circulation 1991; 84(4):1644-1661.
2. Calkins H, Langberg J, Sousa J, et al: Radiofrequency catheter ablation of accessory atrioventricular connections in 250 patients. Abbreviated therapeutic approach to Wolff-Parkinson-White syndrome. Circulation 1992; 85(4):1337-1346.
3. Lesh MD, Van Hare GF, Schamp DJ, et al: Curative percutaneous catheter ablation using radiofrequency energy for accessory pathways in all locations: Results in 100 consecutive patients. J Am Coll Cardiol 1992; 19(6):1303-1309.
4. Kuck KH, Schlüter M: Single-catheter approach to radiofrequency current ablation of left-sided accessory pathways in patients with Wolff-Parkinson-White syndrome. Circulation 1991; 84(6):2366-2375.
5. Lemery R, Talajic M, Roy D, et al: Success, safety, and late electrophysiological outcome of low-energy direct-current ablation in patients with the Wolff-Parkinson-White syndrome. Circulation 1992; 85(3):957-962.
6. Chen SA, Tsang WP, Hsia CP, et al: Catheter ablation of free wall accessory atrioventricular pathways in 89 patients with Wolff-Parkinson-White syndrome—comparison of direct current and radiofrequency ablation. Eur Heart J 1992; 13(10):1329-1338.

7. Schlüter M, Kuck KH: Catheter ablation from right atrium of anteroseptal accessory pathways using radiofrequency current. J Am Coll Cardiol 1992; 19(3):663-670.
8. Lindsay BD, Eichling JO, Ambos HD, et al: Radiation exposure to patients and medical personnel during radiofrequency catheter ablation for supraventricular tachycardia. Am J Cardiol 1992; 70(2):218-223.
9. Calkins H, Niklason L, Sousa J, et al: Radiation exposure during radiofrequency catheter ablation of accessory atrioventricular connections. Circulation 1991; 84(6):2376-2382.

Index

Ablation. See Catheter ablation
Accessory pathways
  radiation exposure in, 217–222
  See also Slow pathway
Action potential prolongation, 13–15
Acute myocardial infarction. See Myocardial infarction
Amiodarone, 169
Antiarrhythmic drugs
  effects on arrhythmia recognition, 140
  effects on defibrillation threshold, 138–140
  and ICD, 137–138, 142–144
  for ventricular tachycardia, 140
Arrhythmia surgery, 177–184
Atrial activation
  during atrial fibrillation, 3–6
  during sinus rhythm, 2
Atrial defibrillation, 31–40
Atrial fibrillation
  activation during, 3–6
  in man, 1–2
  mapping and pacing of, 1–9
  surgical techniques, 180
Atrial flutter, 180

Atrial tachycardia, 180
Atrioventricular nodal reentrant tachycardia (AVNRT), 205, 207, 209–215
Atrioventricular nodal tachycardia, 180–181
Atrioventricular reentry tachycardia (AVRT), 203
AVNRT. See Atrioventricular nodal reentrant tachycardia
AVRT. See Atrioventricular reentry tachycardia

Cardiac arrest, 60–61
Cardiac Arrhythmia Suppression Trial (CAST), 169
CAST. See Cardiac Arrhythmia Suppression Trial
Catheter ablation
  advantages and disadvantages of energy sources, 195–196
  high energy, 189–190
  low energy, 190–191
  principles and techniques, 187–196

radiofrequency, 188, 192–196
  for "Mahaim" tachycardia,
    199–207
  of slow pathway in
    atrioventricular
    nodal reentrant
    tachycardia, 209–215
Computer modeling, of current
    distribution around
    defibrillation electrodes,
    43–55
  data, 45
  experiments, 46–49
  implementation, 46
  structure, 44
Conduction block, 37
Current distribution, 43–55

Defibrillation
  current distribution around
    electrodes, 43–55
  influence of electrode
    position on threshold,
    91–96
  internal atrial, 31–40
  mechanisms of, 25–28
  threshold,
    and antiarrhythmic drugs,
      138–140
    complications of testing,
      110
    definition of, 105–106
    determination of in
      humans, 107–108
    dose–response curves, 106–
      107
    relationship between acute
      threshold and
      therapy outcome,
      110–113
    stability of, 109
  variables influencing, 108–
    109
  See also Implantable
    cardioverter
    defibrillators

Ectopic beats, 19
Electrical stimulation, 166
Electrode(s)
  configurations for atrial
    defibrillation, 31–40
    ideal, 38–39
    research, 40
  current distribution around,
    43–55
  endocardial vs. epicardial, 39
  influence of position on
    defibrillation
    threshold, 91–96
  location and conduction
    block, 37
  location and ventricular
    arrhythmia induction,
    37–38
  polarity, 37
Electrogram patterns, 209–215
Electrophysiology
  of fibrillation, 11–12
  of high voltage shocks, 13–25
    action potential
      prolongation, 13–15
    alteration of activation
      pathway, 19–21
    conduction changes, 16–18
    during fibrillation, 19
    excitability changes, 18
    focal reexcitation, 24–25
    postshock ectopic beats, 19
    synchronization of
      repolarization, 21–24
    tissue damage, 18–19

identifying risk of sudden
death, 61
EMIAT. See European
Myocardial Infarct
Amiodarone Trial
Endocardial electrodes, 39
Epicardial electrodes, 39
European Myocardial Infarct
Amiodarone Trial
(EMIAT), 169–170
Excitability, 140

Fibrillation
electrophysiology of, 11–12
See also Atrial fibrillation;
Defibrillation;
Ventricular fibrillation

High-risk patients. See Patients,
high-risk
Holter facilities, 73–76

ICDs. See Implantable
cardioverter
defibrillators
Idiopathic ventricular
fibrillation, 159–161, 165–
167
Implantable cardioverter
defibrillators
anecdotal data, 73, 76–77
and antiarrhythmic drugs,
137–138, 142–144
basic knowledge about, 67
centers for, 68, 70
choosing, 73–80
and defibrillation threshold,
105–108, 110–112, 114–
115
guidelines for use, 65–70
Holter facilities, 73–76
nonthoracotomy, 119–127

complications, 122–125
overall survival, 125–126
programming, 120–121
spontaneous episodes, 121
therapeutic efficiency, 121–
122
transvenous implantation,
120
patients, 68
for primary electrical disease,
165–167
raw storage data, 74, 80
storage algorithms, 74, 77–80
study of prevention of
sudden cardiac death,
169–175
surgical aspects, 83–90
complications, 87–88
technology, 66–67
transtelephonic monitoring,
149–158
current systems, 151–155
data transmission, 155–156
designs, 156–157
transvenous with pectoral
subcutaneous patch,
99–103
for ventricular tachycardia,
129–136

Leads, 85, 88–89
Left thoracotomy, 83, 84
Left ventricular ejection
fraction, 170, 172
Low gradient region, 20–21

"Mahaim" tachycardia, 199–207
catheter ablation of, 203–207
treatment of, 201–202
Mapping, of atrial fibrillation,
1–9
Median sternotomy, 83–84, 87

Microwave energy ablation, 195–196
MIRRACLEs (Myocardial Infarction Risk Recognition And Conversion of Life-threatening Events), 170
Modeling. See Computer modeling
Myocardial infarction, 57–59, 169–175

National Fund for Scientific Research (NFWO), 172
NFWO. See National Fund for Scientific Research
Nonthoracotomy approach, 85, 88–89, 119–137

Pacemaker-cardioverter defibrillator, 65–70
Pacing
  of atrial fibrillation, 1–9
  termination, 6–9
  rapid, 2
  thresholds, 142
  for ventricular tachycardia in patients with ICD, 129–136
Patients
  high-risk, 57–63
    after myocardial infarction, 57–59, 169–175
    with cardiac arrest, 60–61
    with ventricular tachycardia, 59–60
  and implantable cardioverter defibrillators, 68
  See also specific conditions
Pectoral subcutaneous patch, 99–103
Postshock excitability, 140

Primary electrical disease. See Idiopathic ventricular fibrillation
Programmed electrical stimulation, 166

Radiofrequency catheter ablation, 188, 192–196
  for "Mahaim" tachycardia, 199–207
  radiation exposure of accessory pathways, 217–222
  of slow pathway in atrioventricular nodal reentrant tachycardia, 209–215
Repolarization, 21–24

SAVE. See Survival And Ventricular Enlargement (SAVE) protocol
Sinus rhythm, atrial activation during, 2
Slow pathway, 209–215
Sternotomy, 83–84, 87
Subcostal approach, 84
Subxiphoid approach, 84
Sudden death, 61–63, 169–175
Superior vena cava, 85, 86
Surgery, arrhythmia, 177–184
Survival And Ventricular Enlargement (SAVE) protocol, 172, 173

Tachycardia
  atrial, 180
  atrioventricular nodal, 180–181
  atrioventricular nodal reentrant, 205, 207, 209–215

atrioventricular reentry, 203
"Mahaim", 199–207
See also Ventricular tachycardia
Telephonic monitoring. See Transtelephonic monitoring
Transcoronary ablation, 195
Transtelephonic monitoring, 149–158

U-CARE (Unexplained Cardiac Arrest Registry of Europe), 161–163

Ventricular arrhythmia induction, 37–38
Ventricular fibrillation, 159–161, 165–167, 183
Ventricular tachycardia, 59–60
 antiarrhythmic drugs, 140
 pacing with implantable cardioverter defibrillator, 129–136
 surgical techniques, 181–183

Wolff-Parkinson-White syndrome, 178, 181